F
FOR
FOR

FEEL
30
FOR THE NEXT
50
YEARS

David W. Johnson, Ph.D.

AVON BOOKS NEW YORK

The material in this book is presented for
informational purposes and is not intended to be
a personalized course of treatment. All persons
are advised to consult their own healthcare
practitioners before engaging in any healthcare regimen.

AVON BOOKS, INC.
1350 Avenue of the Americas
New York, New York 10019

Copyright © 1998 by David W. Johnson, Ph.D., and Daniel Klein
Interior design by Kellan Peck
Visit our website at **http://www.AvonBooks.com**
ISBN: 0-380-97463-0

Library of Congress Cataloging in Publication Data:
Johnson, David W. (David Wayne), 1955–
Feel 30 for the next 50 years / David W. Johnson.
        p.   cm.
Includes index.
1. Longevity. 2. Aging. 3. Dietary supplements. 4. Exercise.
5. Nutrition. 6. Stress management. I. Title.
RA776.75.J64   1998   97-53169
613—dc21   CIP

First Avon Books Printing: July 1998

AVON TRADEMARK REG. U.S. PAT. OFF. AND IN OTHER COUNTRIES, MARCA REGISTRADA, HECHO EN U.S.A.

Printed in the U.S.A.

FIRST EDITION

QPM   10   9   8   7   6   5   4   3   2   1

This book is dedicated to new life, present life, as well as to life gone by. The new life is my beautiful infant son Connor, whose loving smile and future expectations give me all the incentive I need to work toward an expanded youthspan. The present life is both my wife Anita, who patiently endured many lost weekends during the writing of this book, and my mother Charlotte, whose own love of life, despite many hardships, never ceases to inspire me. And finally, the past life dedication is for my father Reginald and my brother Kim, who have gone on to be with the Lord. I love and miss you both, and look forward to joining you when my time here is done.

ACKNOWLEDGMENTS

The writing of this book has been an enormous undertaking, and a number of people need to be acknowledged. Daniel Klein, my co-author, was invaluable. A well-published writer, it was Dan who first approached me about producing this book, and once the project was begun, he was able to take my enormous amounts of scientific jargon and massage it into a comprehensive and readable text. I have learned much from him about how a book should be written and how hard it is to "let go" when I have "just one more study that I think should be included." Thanks, Dan.

A special thanks to our agent Howard Morhaim, and the Howard Morhaim Literary Agency in Manhattan, who did an outstanding job of bringing our manuscript proposal to the attention of Avon Books, our publisher. Also, a big thanks to Stephen S. Power at Avon Books for being extremely patient and helpful with this project, prodding me when I needed it, and keeping in the background when he knew I needed more time.

I would also like to acknowledge Gene Giunti, one of my medical students and a registered dietician, for his help in writing the diet section of the book. Also, my chairman in the Department of Physiology at the University of New England's College of Osteopathic Medicine, Dr. Jim Norton, for allowing me to undertake a project of this size, without excess concern that the time input would affect my faculty duties. Furthermore, I would like to thank the personnel in our library for assisting me in my many "Medline" literature searches, particularly Janice Beal and Barb Swartzlander.

Finally, I would like to give a special acknowledgment to my wife Anita for her expert input into the information on internet access, and the use of the World Wide Web to acquire new information. Few know it better.

CONTENTS

Introduction: Staying Young Is the Best Revenge

*E*very Wednesday night in Exeter, New Hampshire, the Over-Thirty Basketball League gathers at the local junior high school gym for a couple of games of ball and, afterward, for a snack at the diner. We are a genial group of hard-working men ranging in age from thirty-two to forty-seven; from an auto-parts salesman to a building contractor to myself, a medical school professor and researcher. One thing we have in common is that we all played sports in high school and college. Another thing we have in common is that we are all terrified of growing old.

Typically, this preoccupation comes out in locker-room jokes and on-court banter. We tease each other about expanding guts and receding hairline, trick knees and failing eyesight. And every now and then one of us will make a joke at his own expense about a memory lapse he experienced just last week, or about how he noticed that his libido is flagging. It is all in fun, but it belies a deep anxiety.

It is not mortality that is on our minds, though—quite the opposite. It is the specter of living old longer, of spending the last quarter of our lives incapable of enjoying ourselves, of losing our memories and our mental acuity, our health, sexuality, and attractiveness. For women, with a life expectancy ten years longer than men, this fear looms even larger.

One Wednesday evening as we were leaving the gymnasium, one of my teammates impulsively blurted out, "God, I'd trade in the last ten years of my life if I could just stay young until the end."

"Actually, you might be able to," I replied. "And you don't have to trade in a day for it."

It was a cold, early winter evening and normally we would have kept to a brisk pace all the way to the diner to avoid getting chilled. But at that moment the entire group came to an abrupt halt and stared at me.

"What are you talking about, Doc?"

"Recent research," I said. "Hormonal-replacement therapies, chronic intake of certain antioxidants, cognitive-enhancing drugs, specific dietary changes, new brain exercises, specific amounts of physical exercise, and stress-reducing visualization techniques that literally convince your body that it is younger—a whole raft of brand-new stuff that can let you stay young well into your seventies, and then some, if you have the willpower to do it."

"You're kidding, right?"

"Nope," I replied. "I see research almost every day that shows we have the capacity to pretty much skip old age. Of course, making this happen takes some real effort, but there's no getting around it—this stuff really works."

I didn't get home until past twelve that night. I had to answer dozens of my basketball league pals' questions, cite research, even write down on place mats and napkins strange-sounding words like "nootropics" (mind-enhancing drugs), proanthocyanidins, and other supplement names like coenzyme Q10, and DHEA. My friends would have kept me there all night if I had not finally gotten away by making them a solemn promise.

This book fulfills that promise. *Feel 30 for the Next 50 Years* details a vast amount of medical research that demonstrates you can extend your brain and body youth well into chronological "old age."

Live Young Longer

I have coined the term Youthspan to mark a sharp distinction with the term "Lifespan." The latter describes the sheer number of years lived, regardless of the quality of those years. Youthspan refers only to the number of years we live in good health, with high energy, strength, and mobility, and with vigorous mental, sensory, and sexual powers.

At the close of the twentieth century, the average Adult Youthspan extends about twenty years, from about age twenty to approximately forty years of age—and then the first signs of progressive and debilitating diseases of old age start to appear. Average Adult Lifespan extends sixty years, from about twenty to eighty years old. Since most of us begin our inevitable decline in optimal health at around age forty, this means we have about forty years with an ever decreasing quality of life to look forward to before we die. *Tripling our Adult Youthspan literally means extending the number of our optimum quality years to sixty—a vigorous and healthy life up to eighty years of age and beyond.*

Obviously, when we extend our Lifespan, we do not necessarily extend our Youthspan. In fact, recent history points to just the opposite outcome. In 1900, the average human life expectancy was about fifty years; now, less than a hundred years later, it is approximately seventy-five years for men, seventy-nine for women—and it is rising fast. But when we only lived to fifty, we did not live through a protracted period of old age; we were not, for example, likely to become senile. It turns out that a host of other diseases were "masked" by this earlier demise, so now as we live a good twenty-five years longer we can expect not only long periods of senility but a host of other debilitating ailments.

Conventional medicine has been little help: all it has basically done is extend our Lifespan so that it is now relatively much longer than our Youthspan. Perhaps the best example of this is what modern medicine has done to deal with the number-one overall cause of death, cardiovascular disease—it has given us coronary bypass and coronary "rotorooter" surgeries, transplant surgeries, clot-dissolving drugs, calcium channel blockers, as well as a host of other pharmaceuticals that keep the old heart beating. This has extended our years of living, but done next to nothing for the quality of our post–heart-attack or post–stroke lives.

Conversely, extending our Youthspan does not necessarily extend our Lifespan—although we are beginning to see evidence that it often does just that. But there is one thing we can be sure of

3

right now: extending our Youthspan can give us triple the number of years of a high-quality, healthy, vigorous, and satisfying life. By following the program in this book, you can radically increase your Youthspan/Lifespan ratio.

YOUTHSPAN—Number of years with . . .

Good Health—*Absence of debilitating diseases associated with aging, including cardiovascular and Type 2 diabetes; "youthful" immune activity and consequent low rate of infection, colds, flu, GI tract illnesses, etc.*

High Energy—*Absence of chronic fatigue associated with aging; not tiring easily or becoming easily fatigued from physical activity.*

Independent Mobility—*Total and unrestricted.*

Full Sensory Acuity—*Eyesight and hearing at full capacity; undiminished sense of taste, hence no consequent loss of appetite.*

High Cognitive Acuity—*Memory, problem-solving ability, verbal agility, etc., all at full, youthful strength; total absence of dementia.*

Full Sexuality—*Libido (sexual desire) and potency at full, youthful strength.*

High Muscle Tone and Strength—*Muscle-to-fat ratio stabilized at youthful level.*

Muscle Control—*Total; absence of involuntary movements, such as tremors.*

Bladder and Bowel Control—*Total.*

Physiognomy: Skin, Hair, Eyes—*Youthful facial appearance; smooth, thick skin tissue; healthy hair; bright eyes.*

LIFESPAN—Number of years with . . .

A Heartbeat—*Quality of those years irrelevant.*

Man Cannot Live by Hormones Alone

The chronic, degenerative, and incurable diseases we acquire in old age actually occur gradually over long periods of time. If you were to be diagnosed with cancer, heart disease, or dementia on your seventy-fifth birthday, it would not have happened overnight—it would be the final result of a process that had been going on in your body for decades. That is why you cannot simply equate good health with "lack of illness." Though you may feel just fine in your youth and middle age, and do not have noticeable symptoms of disease, the cellular processes that will ultimately lead to a full-blown disease in your sixties, seventies, or eighties are now under way.

But the good news is that we can intervene on these decades-long killer processes with various supplements of naturally occurring compounds and synthetic pharmaceuticals, specific changes in our diet, judicious use of brain and body exercises, and some mind-over-body stress-reduction techniques that can dramatically slow the brain and body degeneration that normally occur with age.

Aging is a complex phenomenon that involves, among other things, our endocrine system (hormones) and our immune system (which uses many specific hormones of its own). It encompasses the microdeterioration of our cells and the macrodeterioration of our muscle mass, skin tone, arterial capacity and elasticity, and ultimately organ function. It includes the cellular vitality of our brains and the intrinsic youthfulness of our thoughts and outlook. And whether hormonal or immunological, macro or micro, objective or subjective, the elements that control our Youthspan are fundamentally interdependent—they all feed back to one another.

5

For that reason, my program is comprehensive and interactive. It acknowledges the synergy of hormone and antioxidant supplements with a total calorie- and saturated-fat-restricted diet, and both of these with physical and mental exercise and stress reduction. The documented result of such an all-encompassing program is more than just the sum of its parts, it is a multiple of its parts—supplements multiply the youth-enhancing effects of diet and vice versa.

For example, regular use of either synthetic growth hormone or a growth-hormone release-enhancing compound will very likely increase your muscle-to-fat ratio; yet without the addition of a diet that adequately nourishes these muscles and an exercise program that gives them tone, range, and flexibility, these newly acquired muscles will be of little value to you. But taken all together, each of these elements will enhance the effects of the others. To take another oft-overlooked example, the renewed energy and mental capacity that these supplements and diet can afford you will not mean a thing if you do not adjust your psychological perspective to embrace a Youthspan that is more than twice as long as the one you had originally expected. That means learning how to use and trust your increased memory, how to perceive yourself as young, strong, energetic, and sexy even though according to your birth certificate, "you shouldn't be feeling this way." And perhaps most importantly, it means learning how to enjoy the best of both worlds: the wisdom of experience, and a youthful mind and body with which to use that wisdom.

For these reasons, the Triple-Your-Youthspan Program does not omit any one of the elements of aging or of the various documented strategies for avoiding or reversing aging. Man cannot live on hormones alone—and he certainly cannot extend his Youthspan on them alone, despite the promises made by some of my colleagues in magazine articles and books. I am afraid that the excitement surrounding the discovery of the far-reaching effects of many newly synthesized hormones has caused some eager scientists and supplement-company executives to sound like snake-oil salesmen—a few pills a day will free you from the necessity of watching your diet, maintaining an exercise program, regulating your stress levels, or even giving up smoking. But it just ain't so.

Let me be very clear on this: there is not a doubt in my mind that many of these antioxidants, amino acids, fatty acids, nootropics, and newly available hormones are highly effective at doing their specific jobs when used correctly. They are a large part of what has made it possible for us to radically extend our Youthspan and so, in a sense, really are quite miraculous. But it would be a big mistake to believe that these compounds can do the whole job by themselves. And it would be utter folly to believe that a steady diet of these various supplements will counteract everything else you do to your body. These supplements may be miraculous, but they are not omnipotent!

Two more points about "miracles."

First, there are several antiaging preparations that *appear* very promising at this writing, but which have not, to my mind, been adequately tested for safety and side effects. For example, one promising preparation is L-deprenyl (brand name, Selegiline). In recent years, many studies have shown the use of L-deprenyl to be very effective in alleviating depression and increasing some cognitive functions. For this reason, and because of its safety record, at one point I planned to include L-deprenyl in my program; but recent reports have changed my mind. One of these reports shows that L-deprenyl, when combined with L-dopa in the treatment of Parkinson's disease, actually increases mortality. I have also been seeing information on the Internet stating that some overseas manufacturers of this compound have been marketing an inferior product, in some cases with unacceptable levels of contaminants. So, until more evidence comes in, I cannot in good faith recommend L-deprenyl.

Second, miracle drugs are a growth industry—they probably always have been. Almost daily I receive a catalog or flyer touting the Miracle of the Month—Cat's Claw, the latest crop of blue-green algae, a newly discovered ancient healing tea. The list goes on and on, making it nearly impossible for the average health-conscious consumer to distinguish a truly valuable supplement from one that is, at the very least, insufficiently tested. What happens is a little like Gresham's law in economics wherein valueless money drives good money out of circulation: the plethora of untested miracle health products has a tendency to force the truly remarkable new stuff out of the marketplace, or at least to throw considerable doubt on its efficacy.

Every one of the products advertised in these catalogs may have merit and, as long as they are not harmful, I would fight to the end to prevent the FDA from removing them from the shelves of my health-food store. But as a scientist, I need more than a couple of personal testimonies to believe that they are indeed effective; I need rigorous, controlled, scientific experiments. Of course, I cannot judge next month's miracle drug for you, let alone next year's, so I am also including an appendix on how to access product information and experimental literature on the Internet. There, I will also offer a few general principles for you to use in evaluating this information.

Finally, I wish to assure you that I have no connection, financial or otherwise, with the manufacturers of any of the supplements I recommend in these pages. I wrote this book because, as a medical-school professor, I have become dismayed at the lack of disease-prevention training that occurs in medical schools. We spend almost all our time teaching our doctors how to recognize existing diseases and what drugs or surgery to use to treat them. Even what we call "preventative medicine" in the medical world is, in fact, mostly "catching a disease in its early stages" (with the notable exception of vaccinations). As a result, most physicians will not be able to help you with true disease prevention. But there is hope on the horizon: The American Academy of Anti-Aging Medicine (A4M), founded in 1993, and of which I am a member, represents a growing number of physicians and scientists who are more interested in disease prevention than in disease treatment. One point all of us in A4M advocate is people taking charge of their own health. By the time you are through with this book, you will have much new knowledge to help you in this endeavor. This, I hope, will provide you with the basis for a healthier relationship with your personal physician.

Arrested Development Is a Blessing

Here are the fundamental facts about the well-tested supplements in the Triple-Your-Youthspan Program: a number of recently identi-fied and synthesized critical supplements, primarily antioxidants, fatty acids, amino acids, and hormones, can provide the basis for keeping us younger mentally, emotionally, and physically for a longer time than was ever before possible. Chief among the supplements are the antioxidants, which have the remarkable ability to go directly to the chief cause of cellular aging: free radicals.

Used in conjunction with a healthy diet and exercises, results are often seen and felt almost immediately in increased mental capacity, emotional well-being, greater energy, increased sexuality, and resistance to disease. Both short-term memory and long-term recall increase significantly. Mental agility, perceptual speed, choice reaction time, word fluency, and attention capacity all improve and stay that way as long as the supplements are taken, especially if they are taken along with a program of brain exercises. Emotional problems, such as mood and nonclinical depression, can also be alleviated by these compounds, especially when taken in conjunction with guided mood meditations and stress-reduction exercises.

Fatigue associated with age is also radically reduced, again especially so if complemented with appropriate exercise. Muscular weakness and skeletal fragility are reversed. Resistance to disease, including cardiopulmonary disease and cancer, is significantly enhanced. Also, a significant effect of the program is one's physical appearance. Here, arrested degeneration means maintaining the skin tone, muscles, posture, and carriage of a thirty-year-old well into what used to be called "old age."

The key is that you start the program while you are still relatively young—the way to *stay* young is to *start* young. But even at that, many of you can experience reversal of what little aging has already occurred—particularly in cognitive functions, muscle loss, and immune-system dysfunction.

Staying Young Is the Best Revenge

As a neuroscientist teaching and doing research at the University of New England's College of Osteopathic Medicine, I have designed this program for people over thirty to essentially remain at that age for the next thirty to fifty years of their lives. It is possible to implement my program without going to an expensive longevity clinic here or in Europe. Most of the supplements I recommend are currently available over the counter, although some are easier to come by than others. (I will tell you how to go about getting the hard-to-find ones and how to locate a physician who can prescribe prescription hormones and nootropics.)

The Triple-Your-Youthspan Program is in the vanguard of preventative medicine; in the twenty-first century, these supplements and drugs will be what well-informed people take at breakfast instead of just a vitamin.

CHAPTER ONE

The Biology of Aging

What's He Got That I Don't?

*T*here is nothing quite like a college reunion to get a person thinking about the mysteries of aging.

My God, is that Joe Canty? He looks like he's a hundred and six! What happened to him? Joe was captain of the soccer team and now he looks like he'd pass out if he walked ten yards, let alone jog fifty.

But, over there, isn't that Bob Corey? Or is it his son? No, it's Bob, all right, but he hasn't changed a whit! Look at that full head of hair—not a fleck of gray. And his eyes— clear and bright as a teenager's! And check out that spring in his step as he saunters toward me, a big grin on his unlined face. It's too late to duck him. And it's much too late to do anything about this flabby gut of mine.

The observation we invariably make at these old-school encounters is that some folks age a whole lot faster than others. And among those others are people who appear to barely age at all—not in their physical appearance, not in their apparent strength and endurance, not in their mental sharpness. You do not need to be a molecular biologist to conclude that something (or some things) other than simply the passage of time determines the rate at which we age. And that if we can figure out just what makes Bob Corey "abnormally" youthful while old Joe Canty has one premature foot in the grave, we will be one giant step closer to understanding how to Triple Our Youthspan.

It's All in Your Genes, Right?

There is something strangely comforting in believing that the pace at which we age is totally predetermined at birth, that the clock has been set and wound by Mom's and Dad's (and Grandma's and Grandpa's) DNA, so all we can do is go about our business while the clock runs down to its predestined last tick. Bob Corey lucked out, Joe Canty didn't—that's all She (Mother Nature) wrote.

This is the cold comfort of genetic fatalism. But the reality of what determines how fast we age turns out to be a lot more complicated than that. And high up on the list of complications is the fact that those aspects of our biological setup that control the length of our Lifespan are not necessarily the same as those that control the length of our Youthspan. There are two basic variables that determine how we age:

First, the genetic time clock that governs how long our cells will live if nothing does them any damage. On average, most normal human cells have a good 120 years built into them, which means that if we all lived in Petri dishes under perfectly controlled conditions, we'd live to be about 120 years old.

Second, those environmental forces that damage and kill our cells, via either trauma, toxins, viruses and bacteria, or free radicals. These forces can start doing their dirty work the minute we are conceived and progressively do more damage the longer we live in this perilous, toxin-rich world, recklessly (and inevitably) generating more free radicals as we go along.

In general, there is precious little we can do at this point in medical history to reset our genetic time clock, although, as we will see, there is some fascinating research going on right now that promises to break that barrier. But we do have a great deal of control over the amount of damage our cells incur, both in terms of regulating the number of damaging agents that reach them and in terms of building our resistance to that damage.

The best news is this: Although tinkering with our genetic time clock will primarily have impact only on our Lifespan, controlling cumulative cellular damage during our lives will have a profound impact on Extending Our Youthspan, making our Youthspan the one aspect of aging that we can do something about right now. First, however, let's go over in a little more detail how the body works, so you'll better understand how the Triple-Your-Youthspan Program works.

We're All Prisoners of Our Cells

Our bodies are made of a variety of cells. Some require lots of energy and oxygen to function normally; some require little. Some, such as the epithelial cells lining the intestine, die and replace themselves thousands of times during a person's lifetime. Others, like heart cells and the neurons in the brain, will never divide again after birth. Some have receptors on them that allow them to respond to hormones in the blood like insulin, growth hormone, melatonin, or dehydroepiandrosterone (DHEA), while others do not.

Since all of our organs are made up of cells, when the cells fail, the organ fails. For example, the terms "heart failure" and "heart disease" imply that the heart can no longer effectively pump blood throughout the body, resulting in a person becoming extremely fatigued and unable to do much of anything. But what "heart disease" and "heart failure" ultimately mean is that too many of the cells that make up the heart are not working properly or have just outright died.

This principle applies to all body "failures": to kidney disease, liver disease, and brain disease; to chronic fatigue, failing eyesight and hearing, decreased sexuality, and all the other debilities associated with aging. They all mean that the cells in the relevant organs and systems have failed, or are in the process of failing.

Normal cell death is built into our cells; cell death due to injury is the result of damage via environmental factors, usually either trauma, toxins, infectious agents, or, perhaps most importantly, free radicals.

Normal Cell Death—The Body's Suicide Program

Normal cell deaths occur in our bodies in large numbers all day, every day, often for the purpose of keeping our body in optimal working order. Many types of cells simply "wear out" and are subsequently replaced by the replication of another cell nearby without any net loss to the body. But some cells die and are not replaced, like the abovementioned neurons in our brains that die daily by the millions for an ever increasing net loss.

Cell deaths that are initiated by the body itself are the result of a "suicide program" that is written into the cell's genetic code. Once activated, this program invokes a series of events that instruct the cell to kill itself. Known as a "apoptosis," from the Greek for "falling," biology is loaded with examples of this phenomenon. There are cells in the immune system that will kill themselves after destroying some foreign invader, others that kill themselves to keep an invading virus from replicating itself inside of them and spreading. There are also immune cells which can release chemicals that will initiate the suicide program in another cell's DNA.

But why do cells have a built-in suicide mechanism anyhow? For starters, it protects the body from errant cells. It works like this: if the cell breaks away from the tissue where it belongs and ends up in some other part of the body where it doesn't belong, it will automatically kill itself, thus putting a definitive end to its wandering ways.

Suicide may also keep cells within a tissue from dividing too much. For example, pancreas cells divide in a fetus until they take the form of a normal pancreas, at which point they stop via a suicide program that is then initiated—*Hey, enough is enough, we've got the makings of a nice, functioning pancreas here and we still need room for a few other organs, so stop already!*

Also, if a cell's DNA becomes damaged and is in danger of becoming a cancer cell (a cell that keeps dividing indefinitely), surrounding cells sense the damage and very often will instruct it to kill itself.

But the suicide mechanism can work the other way around too, sending out antisuicide messages, and that is of special interest to those of us who are looking for ways to expand our Youthspan. Consider the embryonic nervous system. When it is developing in a fetus, many neurons will branch out and make contact with other neurons that are just about to kill themselves and send them a signal that says, in effect, *"Don't do it!"*

In recent years, some antisuicide chemical messengers have been isolated by neuroscientists. Clearly one of the future steps for those of us who want to extend our Youthspan is to get these chemicals to tell certain critical, but suicide-prone cells to step back from the ledge.

The suicide and antisuicide mechanisms of neuron cells become particularly relevant when we start thinking about the various forms of dementia that can ruin the last 20 to 25 percent of our lives. Clearly, once a neuron in the brain is gone, that's it—whole neuron files of memories and other functions are erased in the process and not another will appear to replace it. Therefore, our strategy must be to try to decrease the rate at which neurons die or accumulate damage over our lifetimes. And because some types of age-associated dementia seem to kick in when the suicide mechanism of neurons is turned on, we have to do what it takes to reduce their suicide rate.

But suicide is not the only natural cause of cell mortality. Even cells that have a healthy capacity for replicating themselves have a built-in death date, and that is where the Telomere Story comes in.

Normal Cell Death—The Telomere Story

As I write, some of the most dramatic news in the world of the biology of aging revolves around the role and function of telomeres and telomerase. This is the fascinating research that eventually may allow us to actually tinker with our genetic time clocks. Below, I will briefly describe how telomeres work, but let me start by saying this: If ever research offered great promise for an entirely new way to inhibit replicating cancer cells, this is it. And if ever a discovery offered genuine possibilities for radically extending our Lifespan, this one is definitely it too. That's the good news.

The bad news is that if this research fulfills its promise and makes it possible for us to double the durable Lifespan of our cells, the basic end result will be people who live to be 240 years old—with the final 160-plus years of their lives in catastrophic shape!

In other words, lots more Lifespan, but hardly any more Youth-span. That is not very uplifting news for me, folks. Nor for any of my pals in the Over-Thirty Basketball League. But before we get into that, let's return to what exactly telomeres and telomerase are. Telomeres are the ends of chromosomes, which contain important DNA. Normally, small pieces of telomere DNA are lost each time a cell divides, unless the enzyme telomerase prevents this from occurring.

It has been known for some time now that dividing cells can only divide a fixed number of times before they become "senescent." What this means is that, although the cell may be still alive and functional in your body, it no longer has the capability of dividing . . . ever again. Leonard Hayflick demonstrated this back in 1965 when he took living cells from an animal and put them into a culture dish with all the comforts of home and none of the various toxins that can kill cells. Hayflick's cells divided just so many times and then they stopped. Most interesting is the fact that when Hayflick used cells from an old animal in his experiment, they divided fewer times than the same cells from a young animal. His conclusion was that cells in the old animal had already "used up" more of their time-allotted divisions.

This was a sensational finding with regards to aging research, as up to this point scientists believed that all dividing cells could divide indefinitely in a culture dish, as long as you took good care of them. Unfortunately, it was also an example of how scientists refuse to accept new research that goes against dogma; Hayflick could not get his research published in any scientific journals because it was considered too radical. It was not until several other laboratories demonstrated the same phenomenon that scientists finally accepted his research as fact, not fiction.

The evidence became clear: our dividing cells have a built-in clock that is ticking away from the day we are conceived. But exactly what is this ticking clock and where does it do its ticking? The answer appears to be largely due to telomeres, the strands of genetic material at either end of each one of our chromosomes. When a cell divides, becoming two, it must first make a copy of its DNA, which is the genetic material that contains the codes for manufacturing the proteins that make us unique. Almost all of a cell's DNA is stored in the nucleus (over 99 percent of it), with a small amount found in the mitochondria, the cell's power plant (although, as you will see later, this mitochondrial DNA is extremely important). It is the nuclear DNA that is stored in the form of chromosomes—twenty-three matched pairs per cell (with the exception of our sperm and egg cells, and mature red blood cells). Our cells duplicate their nuclear DNA just prior to dividing so that each of the two cells resulting from this division will have a copy.

But each time a cell divides, the telomeres—or tips—of the chromosomes of the new cells become shorter than the telomeres of the chromosomes of the parent cell. This appears to be due to the fact that the enzyme that duplicates the DNA before the cell divides is unable to duplicate the entire length of the telomere strands; it is rather like a Xerox machine that gradually runs out of toner. On and on it goes, the telomeres getting shorter with each replication, until finally they get down to a size where the cell cannot replicate any more. At that point, although the cell is still functional, all it can do is wait to be damaged and to die—it gets the short end, you might say.

The importance of having a population of cells that can divide when necessary is demonstrated in fibroblasts, important cells in our skin that help keep it taut and youthful-appearing. When we are young, fibroblasts are being killed off by the truckload, particularly through excess exposure to sunlight (we tend to spend a lot of time on the beach when we are young). However, when one dies, surrounding fibroblasts sense this and one of them will simply divide into two cells, thus effectively replacing the fibroblast that died with a nice new one. No net loss of cells, and therefore, no visible change in skin appearance in this case. However, once these fibroblasts reach senescence, they will still continue to die due to exposure to sun and exposure to toxins and free radicals generated within the body—the difference is that now they cannot be replaced. The result is the beginning of the appearance of wrinkled skin.

Obviously, these telomere findings are of great interest to cancer researchers. It is clear that cancer cells do not obey normal cell-division laws; instead of eventually dying, they keep on dividing. This suggests that the telomeres in cancer cells are not "shortening unto death" as they do in other cells. Recently, it has been shown that many types of cancer cells contain a rare enzyme called telomerase which seems to repair the telomeres of the chromosomes in the cancer cell after each cell division, so that even after the malignant cell has divided many times, the telomeres have not shortened, giving the cancer cells the dubious blessing of immortality.

Of course, here's where the biologists of aging get very excited: If we could somehow insert the gene which codes for the manufacture of the enzyme telomerase into all of our dividing cells, and these cells then produced telomerase, the telomeres of these cells would not shorten with each successive cell division, and we might be able to significantly increase our Lifespan. But as I cautioned above, before you settle back in your easy chair to wait for the research scientists to figure out how to lengthen your telomeres, you should take careful note of what this discovery would *not* do for you.

Your brain neurons do not divide after birth and consequently do not lose their telomere length (the telomeres of neurons are already quite short at birth from all the dividing they did during fetal development); likewise your heart tissue. So even if there were a "telomere revolution"' that could produce eternally youthful skin and eternally squeaky-clean lungs, you would still be running the same risk of going senile and undergoing heart failure. As youthful-looking as you remained on the outside, you would still be aging considerably on the inside. And even the vainest of us would not trade in an aware-and-awake mind just for great skin.

The Free Radical Theory of Aging

What exactly is it that makes a cell start dividing uncontrollably, resulting in cancer? And what causes our coronary arteries to clog up, resulting in the cells in our heart and blood vessels failing early on, which, in turn, often translates into our suffering through years of cardiovascular disease long before the rest of our body becomes "old"?

Why do our adrenal glands begin to make less and less of the important hormone DHEA over the last forty to fifty years of our life, contributing to a reduction of our libido and producing dysfunction in a number of our physiological systems?

And why do our gonads make less and less testosterone in males and estrogen in females as we age, robbing us of their youth-enhancing properties? Why does our pineal gland start making less melatonin after age forty or fifty, a hormone that we need to help us stay young? Why does our pituitary gland crank out less and less growth hormone in our later years, resulting in our losing muscle and gaining fat, both leading to general frailty?

And perhaps most importantly, why is it that after sixty or more years of life, something goes haywire in certain neurons in our brain, resulting in Alzheimer's disease, or Parkinson's disease?

These are the fundamental questions of aging—the questions whose answers will have the greatest impact on how we extend our Youthspan.

Over the past several years, there have been many basic theories of aging. The Waste Product theory focuses on the fact that cells become less and less able to get rid of their normal wastes as we age, resulting in a surfeit of damaging cellular garbage. The Membrane Hypothesis of Aging concentrates on the damage done to cell membranes over the years that results in the failure of the cell to work properly. And the Theory of Protein Oxidation puts the blame on the proteins inside the cell that become excessively oxidized during aging and eventually kill the cell. Finally, another theory of aging points the finger at the cumulative damage done to our DNA over the years that results in cellular death.

But these days most scientists agree that most, if not all, of the cell damage described by these various theories of aging have one thing in common: they can all be explained by a lifetime of our cells being exposed to various types of free radicals. Therefore, the all-encompassing Free Radical Theory of Aging, first put forth by Dr. Denham Harmon in 1956, is now thought to explain almost all the age-related cell damage that occurs in our bodies.

What exactly is a free radical? Well, our bodies are essentially held together by electrical charges—trillions of negatively and positively charged molecules that ultimately form our bones, skin, muscle, kidneys, brain, and all the rest of us. Our body wants the total number of negative and positive charges to be equal, because atoms and molecules do not like to have a net charge of any type—they want to be neutral.

Our atoms contain a nucleus with several rings of electrons (negatively charged particles) circling around it, usually in pairs. A free radical is simply an atom or molecule that has one or more unpaired or free electrons in its outermost ring. These free electrons make the molecule unstable, meaning that it wants to either give up its free electron to another molecule or take on other electrons which will then pair up with the free electrons; either way it will give the unstable molecule a neutral charge and stabilize it.

The reason these free radicals are dangerous is that when they react with surrounding stable molecules by giving or taking an electron from them, they make these molecules unstable and very often damage them. There are several types of free radicals that our bodies can generate, but there is one type in particular that appears to account for much of the damage to our cells over the years—the oxygen free radical.

Cellular Murders and Oxygen Free Radicals

Oxygen free radicals can kill a cell outright, or they can damage the cell so extensively that the cell will activate its suicide program and do itself in. Either way, it is bad news for us.

Oxygen free radicals are generated from many different sources in our bodies. We are exposed to electromagnetic radiation from the environment all the time (radon, cosmic radiation), and from man-made sources. Some types of electromagnetic radiation can even split water molecules in our bodies to form the very dangerous hydroxyl free radical. This compound only exists for a nanosecond before it attacks whatever molecule is next to it.

One of the chief reasons that oxygen free radicals get to do their damage is because living human beings have this nasty habit of breathing. I am only half joking: Hundreds of well-designed scientific studies have conclusively demonstrated that over time the molecular oxygen we breathe in from our atmosphere results in the formation of some of the most dangerous free radicals in our bodies. Here's how:

The molecular oxygen we suck into our lungs is essential for burning the energy in food and manufacturing cell energy from this process. When carbohydrates, proteins, and fats from our diets are broken down inside our cells, chemical bonds are broken and energy in the form of heat is released. Some of this liberated heat energy (calories) is trapped and transferred into a molecule called adenosine triphosphate (ATP), where it is held until it is needed to build or repair other molecules in the cell.

This process of ATP production occurs only in special structures inside the cell which I mentioned previously—the mitochondria. The mitochondria contain special proteins that are necessary for this process to occur, and many of these special proteins are coded for by the tiny amount of unique DNA that is found in the mitochondria. When particular electrons are created in the mitochondria during the breaking down of the dietary carbohydrates, proteins, and fats, they are grabbed by one of these unique mitochondrial proteins. The mitochondrial protein then hands the electron to the next mitochondrial protein, which in turn transfers it to the next protein, right on down the line like a bucket brigade.

At the end of this line, the last protein hands the electron to the molecular oxygen we breathe, and here is where the electron attaches to it. When the molecular oxygen gains an extra electron, the first commonly generated oxygen free radical is the superoxide anion (SA) free radical. Molecular oxygen needs to accept this electron in order for ATP to actually be made from ADP (adenosine diphosphate); if there was no molecular oxygen to accept this electron, ATP synthesis would halt, our cells would run out of energy in minutes, and we would die. (And that is the basic reason why we have to breathe, no matter how damaging it is!)

When an SA radical then reacts with a stable molecule by either taking an electron from it, or giving it an electron, the free radical itself will become stable after the transaction, but it causes the molecule it reacted with to itself become a free radical. In turn, the new free radical will react in some way with a different stable molecule, causing that molecule to become a free radical, and so on. This "free radical chain reaction" can damage many potentially important molecules in the cell along the way.

Our cells contain an enzyme called "superoxide dismutase" (SOD) that is designed to deal with SA radicals, converting them into less harmful products called peroxides, particularly hydrogen peroxide (yup, the same stuff you keep in your medicine cabinet to put on cuts and scrapes).

However, converting superoxide anions to hydrogen peroxide is not always a good deal. It seems so at first, because you are eliminating the dangerous superoxide anion. Our cells also contain enzymes called "glutathione peroxidase" (GPX) and "catalases" (CAT) that normally break down the hydrogen peroxide molecule—

which is not itself a free radical—back into water and molecular oxygen. This is all well and good, as it results in the elimination of hydrogen peroxide from the body. This entire process can be seen in the figure below:

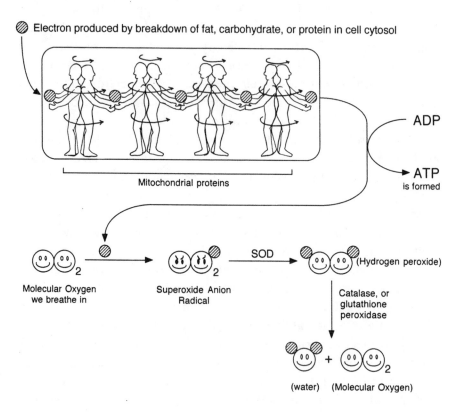

However, before it can be destroyed by GPX or CAT, some of the hydrogen peroxide generated from the SOD neutralization of SA free radicals goes on to react with free metal ions (such as iron and copper) in the cells. It can also react with certain metal ions present in proteins in the cell that act as enzymes. This process is known as the Fenton reaction and it results in the formation of the extremely damaging hydroxyl free radical:

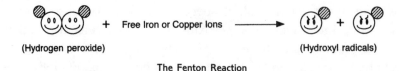

The Fenton Reaction

The hydroxyl radical then attacks and damages any cell structures around it. If it happens to attack nearby proteins, this results in the creation of substances scientists can measure, called carbonyl compounds. It is now well known that these carbonyl compounds accumulate with age in mammalian cells, especially our brain cells, and animal studies demonstrate that the accumulation of carbonyl compounds in brain cells is positively correlated with decreased cognitive function.

Our bodies have essentially no defense against the hydroxyl radical, other than to minimize its production. Therefore, this ability of free iron to react with peroxides and generate hydroxyl radicals is the reason that high levels of total body iron in older adults are now thought to be harmful to our Youthspan (a fact which I discuss later in Chapter 16). And this is why we have to do what we can to minimize our levels of total body iron as we get older.

DNA Damage by Oxygen Free Radicals

Death of our cellular mitochondria due to oxygen free radical damage to our mitochondrial DNA has become an entire field of medicine. In fact, it is now believed that over a hundred different age-related diseases are due to primary defects in the mitochondria within specific types of cells such as neurons, muscle cells, and heart cells.

Because we make such a large amount of damaging SA free radicals daily in our mitochondria, and because many of them end up ultimately being transformed into the much more dangerous hydroxyl free radical, the mitochondrial DNA along with the cell membranes in the mitochondria take a big oxygen-free-radical hit over the years. Eventually, the mitochondrial DNA can become so damaged that the mitochondria are no longer able to make the proteins that are needed for life-sustaining ATP synthesis and the cell dies.

Science has provided us with lots of evidence for mitochondrial-mediated cell death via oxygen free radicals. For example, if you put an animal under increased oxidative stress (meaning more oxygen free radicals than normal are produced), the DNA gets damaged. We know this because we can measure a substance in the urine called 8-OHDG (8-hydroxydeoxyguanosine) that is produced when DNA is repairing itself after it gets damaged.

Compounding the problem, it appears that as our cells get older, their DNA becomes even less capable of handling an above-average dose of free radicals. In fact, if you compare old human cells and young human cells in laboratory dishes under identical oxidative stress conditions, the older human cells crank out four times as much 8-OHDG as the younger cells. In a word, there's a lot more damage occurring.

So the lesson is clear: *the older we are, the more important it is to start doing what we can to get our oxidative stress under control.*

Cell Membrane Damage by Free Radicals

The special cell membranes within the mitochondria itself are not the only ones that get damaged by free radicals. The cell membrane surrounding the entire cell also takes a big hit. The cell membrane is primarily made up of different types of fats and lipids (fattylike substances, like cholesterol), and these lipids are the constant targets over the years of oxygen and other types of free radicals.

What seems to happen during this process is that the hydrogen peroxides and other peroxides formed from SOD neutralizing the SA radicals can react with the polyunsaturated fats which are among the major components of our cell membranes. This reaction, called lipid peroxidation, links together the fats in our cell membranes and makes what was once a nice, soft, gelatinous cell membrane much more rigid. Not good news, since a soft, gelatinous cell membrane is needed for things to pass in and out of the cell in proper amounts. We know this reaction occurs because it ultimately results in the formation of compounds such as lipofuscin, which we can measure in cells.

Some scientists have suggested that lipofuscin itself is not a particularly harmful molecule, but as the Hungarian physician Imre Zs. Nagy first posed in 1978, accumulations of it are an excellent marker that adverse age-related changes are occurring in cell membranes. And sure enough, when we look at the cell membranes in older animals, we see a lot more of it than in young animals, especially in cells in the central nervous system, including the human nervous system. In fact, lipofuscin is the pigment that produces the so-called liver spots on the skin in the elderly.

I find it very interesting that age-related excess protein oxidation has been reversed in animals. One such study demonstrated that old gerbils have nearly twice as much oxidized protein in their brain cells as young gerbils, and that the old gerbils also have deficits in certain types of memory, exemplified by their poor performance (compared to young gerbils) in what is called a radial arm maze test. However, when the old gerbils were chronically treated with a potent, synthetic antioxidant called PBN [phenyl-tert-butyl-nitrone] (not yet available for people) the amount of oxidized protein in their brain was decreased. Now, when these PBN-treated old gerbils were tested in the radial arm maze, their performance was as good as the young gerbils. Fascinating stuff.

The Body's Dumb Short-Range Planning

First, it was breathing: We can't live without doing it, but by breathing we generate oxygen free radicals that slowly age us. Unfortunately, our immune system sticks us with a similar, can't-win-for-losing scenario.

This phenomenon occurs when chronic inflammation, such as chronic viral or bacterial infections, causes specialized immune cells to go after the foreign invader. Many of these immune cells produce oxygen free radicals to help destroy the foreign invader; this protects against the immediate danger of the invader, but the free radicals themselves can also damage the DNA and cell membranes of healthy cells in the area. This, in turn, may either kill the cells or damage the cells, increasing the chance that they will mutate and possibly even become cancerous. Hey, thanks for all the help, guys.

Another critical source of destructive free radicals is a series of enzymes known as cytochrome P-450 that are mostly contained in liver cells. Their major function is to destroy toxic chemicals that enter our body daily through our water, air, or food. Once again, when these enzymes are activated, they deal with the clear and present danger by destroying the invading foreign chemicals. Again, nice work, fellas, except for one little problem: this very act produces free radicals which, in the long run, damage the same cells that produce them.

The only conclusion we can draw from all of this is that the human body is ultimately a victim of its own, short-term planning.

Free Radicals—The Body Fights Back . . . Badly

Our bodies basically have three ways to protect us from the inevitable production of these free radicals:

First, they savor the antioxidants present in some of our foods, like the flavonoids, vitamins E, C, and the carotenoids.

Second, our bodies manufacture certain molecules that act as antioxidants; some of the most studied of these are glutathione, alpha lipoic acid, uric acid, and the hormone melatonin.

And third, our cells have built-in antioxidant defense enzymes they synthesize for their war against free radicals. Three of these systems are extremely important, and I mentioned them briefly above: superoxide dismutase (SOD), different types of which require minerals like manganese, copper, or zinc as cofactors to function normally; glutathione peroxidase (GPX), which requires the mineral selenium as a cofactor to function properly; and the catalases (CAT). As you saw above, the role of both GPX and CAT is to take the hydrogen peroxide and other peroxides that are formed when SOD neutralizes the SA free radicals, and to destroy them.

How important are these built-in antioxidant enzymes in fighting off and neutralizing dangerous oxygen free radicals? Researchers have shown that if you give common house flies extra copies of the genes which have the genetic codes for both SOD and the catalases, they not only will live up to one-third longer than flies without the extra copies, they will experience a much-delayed loss in physical performance!

In the fly universe, this means being able to buzz around like a youngster well into "old age" (three days old). In ours, it means an extended Youthspan to accompany an extended Lifespan—the ideal outcome!

More recent research has found that creating strains of rats with fewer copies of the genes for some of these antioxidant enzymes results in these mammals suffering from all sorts of problems in their nervous and cardiovascular systems, related to free radical damage. In addition, scientists studying aging sometimes use an animal model called the "senescent-accelerated mouse" (the 'SAM' mouse). This mouse grows old and dies much earlier than most mice. Recently, it was shown that one of the reasons for this is that this animal has inadequate levels of SOD in its mitochondria.

Along these same lines of science, a recent long-term study of male and female macaque monkeys followed over a 4.5-year period found that the antioxidant status of these monkeys (measured by monitoring plasma levels of seven antioxidant compounds, including vitamins C, E, and the carotenoids) was negatively correlated with their "rate of biological aging." In other words, the monkeys that maintained the highest blood levels of antioxidants over these years aged more slowly and got less disease than monkeys which had chronically lower levels of plasma antioxidants. Just more and more evidence indicating that if we don't do what we can to minimize free radical production in our bodies, it appears we will age and acquire disease more quickly.

CHAPTER TWO

The Free-Radical Hit List

*L*et's take several steps up the micro-macro ladder and take a look at how some of our tissues are affected by chronic exposure to free radicals. This hit list will demonstrate just a few of the disorders known to be due to free radicals, and how much the Youthspan crisis is the result of free radicals wreaking havoc with our aging bodies.

Unfortunately, it is not a pretty sight.

The Immune System

It has been known for years that "normal" aging is associated with a gradual decline in the functions of our immune system. Therefore, the way things stand now, the longer we live, the weaker our immune systems become. And this weakness begins distressingly early: the incidence of infectious diseases such as pneumonia and influenza rises exponentially after age twenty-five! There are similar statistics for digestive problems, skin rashes, urinary tract infections— the whole list of age-associated infectious diseases. Not only do we run into trouble with our normally "friendly" microbe population as we get older, we also become less efficient at detecting and dealing with new foreign microbes that we bring into our bodies through the air we breathe and the food and water we consume. In fact, this is thought to be one of the principal reasons why we are increasingly more likely to develop cancer as we age. It is even difficult to vaccinate the elderly, as their immune systems may not be able to generate enough antibodies to the vaccine to provide them any protection against the disease for which they are being vaccinated. Clearly, a compromised immune system is not conducive to a long Youthspan.

Many different types of specialized cells form a coordinated attack unit in a healthy immune system. But, unfortunately, the DNA of these critical immune cells provides a good target for oxygen free radicals. Much of the evidence demonstrating this comes from studies of two of the immune system's most potent cells, the B- and T-cells; both are markedly inhibited when exposed to oxidizing compounds. Fortunately, it has been shown that some of these adverse effects on immune cells produced by oxidizing compounds can be reversed in elderly people, simply by taking oral antioxidants. For example, it was recently shown by Dr. Simin Meydani and others at the Nutritional Immunology Laboratory at Tufts University that supplementing elderly persons with 200 milligrams daily of the potent antioxidant vitamin E for just four months improved the immune response to diphtheria and tetanus vaccines. This is a very important finding for those elderly who do not respond well to vaccines. In addition, Dr. Michelle Santos of the Jean Mayer USDA Human Nutrition Research Center on Aging at Tufts University showed that years of taking fifty milligrams on alternate days of the potent antioxidant beta carotene increased the activity of natural killer cells (immune cells that actively seek out and destroy newly formed cancer cells) in older men.

Cancer

Cancer may be the most preventable disease that shortens our Youthspan. But before I proceed to tell you why, I need to be perfectly clear about the distinction between early cancer detection and the actual prevention of cancer. Much of what is done in your doctor's office revolves around the early detection of cancer: PAP smears, breast and testicular examinations, mammograms, evaluation of skin lesions, digital prostate exams, sigmoidoscopies, etc. This is great because there is certainly a much improved prognosis if you catch this disease before it has spread from its site of origin.

However, if you are a person in whom this disease is caught early, you still have something in common with the person in whom the disease is caught late: *you both have cancer.* Although your prognosis will be much better, you are still going to become a part of the cancer establishment; you will suddenly find yourself shunted to the oncologist's office where you might be told you need surgery, radiation therapy, or a regimen of chemotherapy just to make sure no wandering cells have escaped. All of this results in a greatly increased stress level, which itself is harmful to your Youthspan.

It is now believed that about 90 percent of all cancers are caused by substances in our environment (including our diet) doing damage to our DNA over long periods of time, which subsequently can affect the cell cycle clock, the proteins that regulate cell growth. This cumulative DNA damage can come from multiple environmental sources, including the carcinogens and mutagens in cigarette smoke, pesticides, certain hormones, toxins found in variable amounts in both plants and meat, excessive saturated fats in our diets, various pollutants in our air and water, and excessive alcohol intake. All of these things have something in common—they can generate lots of free radicals within our bodies, causing damage in our DNA. Therefore, it is believed by many scientists that it is ultimately free radical damage to DNA that is a major cause of many cancers.

Some of the proof for this comes in the epidemiological evidence, which shows a strong inverse relationship between consumption of foods rich in antioxidants and the incidence of cancer. Studies which follow healthy people over years have consistently demonstrated that those people with chronically lower plasma levels of antioxidants are more likely to develop various types of cancer. In fact, in his CD-ROM on the prevention and therapy of cancer, Dr. Charles Saunders, a noted expert on the causes of cancer at both the University of Washington and Washington State University, cites several studies of carotenoid intake and cancer. Some of these studies show a significantly reduced risk of cancer in the lung, breast, cervix, stomach, oral cavity, pharynx and urinary bladder in those people with the highest intake of carotenoids such as beta carotene.

The reason that antioxidants seem to be effective in preventing cancer from occurring is that the process of a cell going from normal to cancerous appears to require several steps over several years— probably decades—to occur. In fact, the progression from normal to precancer and then to cancer cell is well established in all multistep experimental carcinogenesis models. This means that there is a vast window of time in which to do things that may prevent a "precancerous" cell from progressing all the way to a true cancer. One of these things is chemoprevention (not to be confused with "chemotherapy"—the use of toxic drugs to treat existing cancer). This is the systemic use of specific natural or synthetic agents to reverse or arrest a premalignant cancer cell before it can progress to a malignant and invasive cancer. High on the list of these agents are antioxidants.

Cataracts

Most people over the age of sixty develop cataracts, which is a clouding of the lens in the eye. As a result, light is not focused properly on the retina in the back of the eye, and the affected person experiences blurry vision.

Cataracts were once one of the scourges of aging—the beginning of the end. But today surgery for cataract removal has been honed to an art form—patients getting this procedure can be in and out of the hospital in only a few hours. Presently, cataract surgery is the most common surgery in the United States, with over one million operations being performed each year. Of course, there is the usual catch: this little bit of surgery costs the health-care system over three billion dollars annually.

But it turns out that costly, after-the-fact surgery is not the only solution to the cataract problem. A large amount of scientific evidence now suggests that the gradual development of cataracts is just one more age-related problem that we can chalk up to free radicals. At least five epidemiological studies have shown that vitamin C, vitamin E, and the carotenoids have strong preventive effects on cataracts. The take-home lesson from all this appears to be that when a person increases the amount of oxidative stress he is under—say, by smoking—he multiplies his risk for developing cataract development. And increasing antioxidant intake either through dietary means or supplements, or both, can prevent this disorder.

Cardiovascular Disease

Cardiovascular disease remains the number-one cause of death in this and most other developed countries. In the past twenty to thirty years, we have managed to develop an increasing number of exotic and invasive ways to postpone death from cardiovascular disease— one of the main reasons why the average lifespan has increased so much in this century. However, the quality of life for people with significant cardiovascular disease often leaves much to be desired; nothing will shorten your Youthspan faster than a chronic cardiovascular problem. Here again, prevention of the disease in the first place is far preferable to treatment of an existing disease.

What role do oxygen free radicals play in cardiovascular disease? A long line of evidence now shows that when molecules of the "bad" type of cholesterol (low-density lipoprotein or "LDL") are attacked by free radicals, the LDL molecule is oxidized to a form that is far more easily taken up by the cells lining the walls of our arteries. Thus begins the dreaded disease atherosclerosis, wherein a plaque of fatty material pushes out from the wall of the artery, blocking the flow of blood. As a result, all the tissue downstream of the block loses most or even all of its blood supply and is injured or dies; when this happens in the coronary arteries, it can result in a heart attack. It is now well established that the use of antioxidants, particularly vitamin E, can prevent the oxidation of LDL, and thus prevent coronary-artery disease from occurring.

Brain Aging

When it comes to free radical damage, the brain is a sitting duck. It cannot win for losing—and what we are losing is brain cells. The result is everyone's worst fear: age-associated dementia.

As I've mentioned, neurons cannot replicate themselves if they become damaged or die. On top of this, neurons get bombarded by loads of oxygen free radicals throughout a person's life. This is because neurons have a particularly high rate of metabolism, which means they produce many more oxygen free radicals than other tissues in our bodies. It would seem reasonable to expect the body to be prepared to counter this surfeit of brain-born free radicals with a well-fortified antioxidant defense system complete with loads of SOD, glutathione peroxidase, and catalase. But, sadly, this is not the case: Brain cells actually have relatively low concentrations of these important antioxidant defenses compared to other body cells.

When we compare the brains of old animals with those of young animals, we almost always see that older brain cells have much more lipofuscin in them, primarily the result of cumulative free radical damage occurring over the lifetime of the animal.

And there is growing evidence that mitochondrial-mediated cell death is a major factor in the onset of neurological diseases of many types. For example, a recent study by Dr. Marisol Corral-Debrinski from the Department of Genetics and Molecular Medicine at Emory University School of Medicine found a significant increase in mutations in mitochondrial DNA taken from neurons in certain parts of the brain of elderly people. The author concluded that these mutations in mitochondrial DNA in older brains might contribute to the neurological impairment associated with aging. Indeed, when physicians examine the mitochondrial DNA of people who already have neurodegenerative diseases such as Alzheimer's, Parkinson's, and Lou Gehrig's disease, they often find mutations in the mitochondrial DNA, probably caused by decades of overexposure to free radicals.

Saving our brains, then, is a formidable problem, one whose solution is necessary if we are to have an extended Youthspan.

CHAPTER THREE

No Brainer

*F*or most of us, the image of growing old badly means first and foremost losing mental function. This fear outstrips all others— even our fear of loss of mobility. We might be able to tolerate spending the final years of our lives in a wheelchair, but not without a reliable memory, without the capacity to absorb information, without the ability to think or talk about anything but the immediate present, without the thoughts and feelings that make us who we each are. And this fear rears its ugly head the first time we realize we cannot remember a once-familiar telephone number or where we parked our car. That moment is often in our early forties. And now medical science has made it possible for us to outlive our brains by decades.

Let's take a more detailed look at how the brain works and why it loses function as it ages. In this way, we will be better able to understand how the various supplements and lifestyle adjustments I will soon tell you about can protect and maintain your cognitive abilities. In short, how we can actually keep our brains young, healthy, and bright along with the rest of our bodies.

How the Healthy Brain Works

There are essentially two major types of cells in the brain, neurons and glial cells. Neurons are the cells in the brain that transmit information from one part of the brain to other parts of the brain or from the brain to other organs. Glial cells can be thought of as the support staff for our hard-working neurons; they are absolutely essential for keeping the neurons nourished. The cell body of the neuron extends out at several different points, forming structures called dendrites. The cell body is also where the nucleus resides, the home of the neuron's DNA. The axon of the neuron is usually sheathed with a substance called myelin that acts as an electrical insulator, allowing the neuron to send electrical signals more effectively. The terminal boutons, or "tips" of the neuron, contain packages called vesicles which contain the chemical neurotransmitter that the neuron uses to communicate with other neurons. A typical neuron looks like this:

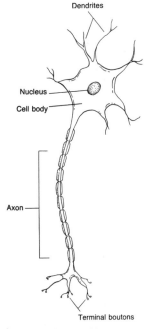

The "Typical" Neuron

Neurons are densely packed together in the brain. When the terminal boutons of one neuron push up against the dendrites and cell body of a neighboring neuron, they are separated by a tiny gap called a "synapse." Thus, in neuroscience jargon, when terminal boutons of one neuron push up against the cell bodies and dendrites of other neurons, we say those terminal boutons are *synaps-*

ing on those dendrites and cell bodies. The neuron that is projecting the terminal boutons into the synapse is called the "presynaptic" neuron, and the neuron whose dendrites and cell body are synapsing with those terminal boutons is called the "postsynaptic" neuron:

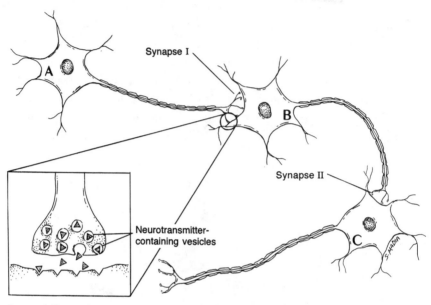

Synapse I: Neuron A is presynaptic to Neuron B. Synapse II: Neuron C is postsynaptic to Neuron B.

When a presynaptic neuron fires, that is, releases its neurotransmitters into the synapse, these chemicals quickly travel across the synapse and bind to special receptors on the dendrites and cell body of the postsynaptic neuron. This often results in the postsynaptic neuron becoming "excited," and if it gets excited enough, it will also fire. This electrical action spreads along the postsynaptic neuron from where it originated in the cell body down to the axon and its terminal boutons. When the impulse arrives at the terminal boutons, it stimulates the release of the neurotransmitters stored there into the next synapse down the line. Often a single nerve will have dozens—even hundreds—of surrounding neurons forming synapses with it. Some of the neurotransmitters these nerves release into the synapses excite the neuron; others may inhibit it from becoming excited. When a neuron gets a bunch of contradictory messages, it takes a poll: If the majority of signals are excitatory, it will fire; if the majority are inhibitory, it won't. Very democratic, these neurons.

The neurons in our brain are releasing neurotransmitters in different parts of our brains millions of times each second, either causing other neurons to fire or to not fire. Sometimes causing a group of neurons to fire will get the wanted result, such as processing a memory into long-term storage, and sometimes causing neurons to not fire will get the result you want, such as sitting still. The bottom line is this: these millions of neurons that are firing and not firing each second are doing so through the release of neurotransmitters into synapses, and when we age and get age-related neurological diseases, neurons develop all kinds of problems in releasing their neurotransmitters when they should. When this happens, some neurons in some parts of the brain may start firing when they really should be quiet, and neurons in other parts of the brain may remain quiet when they really should be firing. (Of course, if the neurons simply die, whatever role they played in maintaining normal brain function is lost.)

Synaptic Vacuuming

Not only is it important to maintain a relatively stable number of synapses over our lifetimes for our brains to age successfully, but the synapses must be functional as well. And one of the most important things that occurs in a synapse that is working properly is that the neurotransmitters released into that synapse are removed very quickly. The reason for this is fairly simple. Once a neurotransmitter is released into a synapse, it will travel across it and bind to its receptor on the postsynaptic neuron in just a few thousandths of a second. If the neurotransmitter is allowed to stay in the synapse for even just a few seconds, it can overstimulate the postsynaptic neuron and produce all sorts of neurological problems. Therefore there are a number of mechanisms our brain employs to remove neurotransmitters from synapses quickly after they have been released.

One way is through the use of special "re-uptake pumps" on some terminal boutons that essentially suck up the neurotransmitter that was released and pump it right back into the neuron that released it in just milliseconds. Then that neuron can actually recycle the neurotransmitter and release it again in the future. Another common way to remove neurotransmitters from a synapse is through special enzymes present in the synapses that quickly bind to the neurotransmitter after it is released and break it down into harmless components. Both of these vacuuming techniques can become less effective as our brain cells age and die. They need a little extra help from us. Happily, as we will see, help is on the way in the form of hormone supplements, nootropic drugs, and antioxidants.

Neuronal Pathways and Neurological Disease

Neuronal pathways are basically clusters of billions of neurons whose cell bodies all originate in one part of the brain and whose axons project to some other part of the brain, forming synapses with other neurons. Some neuronal pathways are important in hearing, seeing, and smelling; others are important in motor functions; and still others are critical in forming memories.

Thus, when we get a disease that specifically affects the neurons in a certain neuronal pathway, the function of that specific pathway will be compromised. You do not need to be a neuroscientist to recognize that Alzheimer's disease predominantly targets neurons in the neuronal pathways that are responsible for some types of memory, personality, mood, and to some extent, motor function. Similarly, Parkinson's disease predominantly kills brain neurons in pathways involved in regulating our motor functions.

When it comes to lengthening Youthspan, our major concerns are those parts of our brain that perform cognition. Cognition includes all aspects of perceiving, learning, thinking, and remembering, and is not only the stuff of consciousness, but also the basis of personality. If you cannot remember your experiences, you have no personal history; and if you have no personal history, you cannot feel like a complete person.

Remember This!

In the upper, more advanced parts of our brain are found the association areas of the neocortex. These areas are believed to be responsible for initially processing the information that comes to us via what we see, hear, smell, and touch, and it is here the information is temporarily stored in the form of short-term memories. From there it can be shuttled to long-term storage (memory in short-term storage that is not transferred to long-term storage will eventually be lost). The part of the brain most important in long-term memory is the limbic cortex, which contains the hippocampus, a structure that enables us to manage and encode long-term storage memories. It is during the time that short-term memory is being processed for long-term memory storage that it is most vulnerable to being erased.

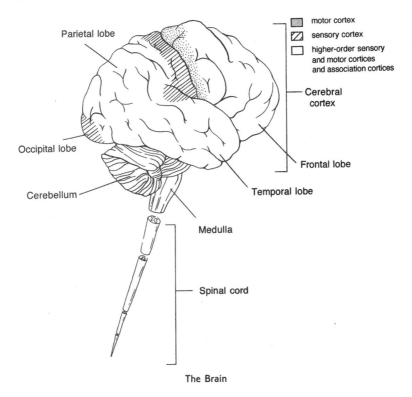

The Brain

A good example of this is the effect of trauma on short-term memory. A person who gets a concussion playing football often cannot remember how he got his injury—the thoughts that were stored in his short-term memory at the time of the trauma have been erased by the trauma. However, these people rarely have problems with their long-term memories when they recover from these insults to their brain. In fact, it is quite common to read in medical journals about patients with severe concussions who cannot remember events occurring several days prior to the concussion (retrograde amnesia), yet their long-term memory is perfectly intact. In addition, people undergoing surgery are often given drugs that will interfere with their ability to process memories, and they therefore will remember little or nothing about the surgery afterwards (even if they were mildly conscious).

Those of you who are familiar with computers may start to see some correlations between human memory and some of the functions of your computer. On your computer's "hard-drive," information is permanently stored on magnetic disk. However, when you want to recall information out of your hard drive, you have to first transfer a copy of it to the random access memory (RAM) of your computer, where you can then use it or manipulate it. Therefore, RAM is somewhat analogous to the association areas of the cerebral cortex, and the hard drive is similar to the hippocampus.

Putting information into your computer is also somewhat similar to putting information into your brain. On the computer, the incoming information is first entered into some software program, which is using RAM memory. However, this information must be saved, so it is stored on your hard drive to keep it from being erased. As all computer users know, information processed using your RAM memory is usually gone for good if there is a power surge or power loss before you can save this information on your hard drive—thus the analogy I used above describing how trauma can erase short-term memory if it has not yet been filed away in long-term memory.

Your Brain Has Potential

A complex phenomenon known as "long-term potentiation" (LTP) helps explain how we form long-term memories. And we need some knowledge of it in order to understand why certain diseases like Alzheimer's can destroy long-term memories, and why certain so-called smart drugs are able to enhance memory formation and learning.

It starts with synapsing. When we form long-term memories, part of what happens is that the presynaptic neurons bringing information about recent memories into the hippocampus from other parts of the brain form synapses with postsynaptic neurons within the hippocampus itself. Many of these presynaptic neurons release a neurotransmitter called glutamic acid into the synapse, which in turn binds to receptors called "NMDA" (N-methyl-D-aspartate) receptors on the postsynaptic neurons and stimulates them to fire. Interestingly though, when a large number of these hippocampal neurons are stimulated to fire, they then keep on firing for days, weeks, even months without further stimulation. This continuous firing is "long-term potentiation," and when LTP occurs, it somehow alters the structure of the synapse, allowing long-term memories to be placed into the hippocampus for storage. In short, our long-term memories result from the release of certain chemicals into synapses in the hippocampus. So, any disease or breakdown that affects the hippocampus is going to have adverse effects on our long-term memory functions.

Since these NMDA receptors seem to be so important in forming and storing long-term memories, studies have been undertaken to see if the levels of these receptors change during the normal aging process. The results strongly suggest that, yes, the density of these receptors in the brains of mammals, particularly in the hippocampus, decreases considerably with age. Part of the reason for their decrease may be due to the receptors being oxidized by free radicals. In fact, several animal studies have demonstrated that administration of potent antioxidants such as alpha lipoic acid can prevent oxidation of NMDA receptors in the brain—in some cases even reverse some of the NMDA receptor deficits. This, in turn, is correlated with an increase in cognitive function in these animals.

How Much Do You Have to Forget Before Medicine Remembers You?

The evidence is pretty clear: "Normal" aging has a gradual but direct debilitating effect on our brains, and a major reason for this is the cumulative damage done by free radicals over the years. So, for example, even people who are healthy and in more-or-less full possession of their cognitive marbles when they reach the age of sixty-five have many more mutations in the mitochondrial DNA of their brain cells than do young people. They've accumulated them simply by living longer. And, if they live long enough, they will probably accumulate enough of these mutations to finally have a neurological disease.

This is the basis of a new research model of dementia known as the "threshold model." It basically says that your brain has some amount of cognitive "reserve" which allows you to keep your cognitive functions intact even if damage is accumulating in your brain over the years. However, once the amount of functional brain damage reaches some critical "threshold" level, the signs and symptoms of dementia start to appear. One day you're healthy, one day you're not. But this model doesn't mean we're helpless; instead it offers hope. For if neurological disease does indeed occur over long periods of time, then many age-related diseases of the brain appear to have large "windows of opportunity" during which we can intervene earlier in life, before they can progress to become irreversible problems.

So rather than wait until I acquire some form of dementia, then work with my doctor to try to maximize whatever memory and other cognitive functions I have left, I want to know right now how to prevent the gradual onset of damage to the cognitive-functioning areas of my brain. And to this end I have turned to the burgeoning scientific evidence that implicates the long-term use of antioxidants, antiinflammatories, caloric restriction, physical exercise, stress-reduction therapies, and estrogen-replacement therapy in women for protecting their brains from neurological disease, particularly the one most feared of all, Alzheimer's.

There is one more thing we can do to keep our brains young—frequent mental exercises throughout our lives to promote "synaptic plasticity." Here's how that works:

Synapses are not stable entities; they can actually change their form. The physical size of a synapse can be modified when neurons alter their communication level with each other; it can become bigger or smaller, thereby changing the effectiveness of whatever message that particular area of the brain transmits. This ability to "remodel" synapses is synaptic plasticity, and it is the key to the "use it or lose it" phenomenon. As a result of synaptic plasticity, if neurons in a certain pathway die in large numbers, the surviving neurons can modify their synapses with the next neurons they contact downstream, making a more effective connection—they pick up the slack for the dead neurons.

Now it turns out that simply inputting information to form memories alters the structure of many of our brain synapses—in short, giving the brain work to do promotes synaptic plasticity. Several large studies of middle-aged and older people now conclusively demonstrate that those who spend more time in school pursuing an education (which implies more memorizing and processing information than that done by people who do not pursue education) have a significantly lower risk of getting dementia when they are older, particularly Alzheimer's disease. As a child I never would have believed it: school is good for your health.

CHAPTER FOUR

The Young Brain/Young Mind/
Young Body Cycle

*To understand why warts disappear if you receive a hypnotic
suggestion (or if you wash your hands in moonlight), we must
break down some of the existing divisions in knowledge.*

—ANNE HARRINGTON,
Harvard University historian

Stress and the Human Condition

*I*n the early part of this century, a young Austrian physician
named Hans Selye found that when he injected different types of
extracts into animals, they developed certain common symptoms, including enlargement of the adrenal cortex, gastrointestinal ulcers, and
shrinkage of the lymph nodes. He was surprised at their commonality
because the compounds he injected were quite different from one
another.

He then realized that the common denominator in his experiment was that all the animals were getting injections, regardless of
what extract was being injected. He began noting that the animals
did not like being injected with a needle and would struggle to
avoid the injections. It was then that he realized that it was the
"stress" (which he defined as the non-specific response of an organ-
ism to a demand made upon it) of the injection itself, not what was
in the syringe, that caused these common symptoms of illness.

Later, Selye found that every creature he studied had some type of characteristic stress reaction to change in its internal or external environment whether that was being injected with some compound, or being exposed to excess heat or cold, pain, muscular work, or simply loud noise. If this stress reaction was maintained for a long enough period of time, the animal subjects became ill. Dr. Selye demonstrated that just about every living creature has some set of standard biological responses it uses to deal with different types of stress—and that definitely includes human beings. Selye's studies were the beginnings of the wealth of knowledge we have today on how stress makes us ill and depressed, and how it robs us of a long and healthy Youthspan.

What Grandmother Knew

Recently, a number of high-profile physicians have created a veritable cottage industry based on a piece of knowledge that not only Hans Selye knew, but virtually everybody's grandmother also knew: Our mental states profoundly affect our physical states. Or, as my grandmother used to put it, "Stop being so nervous or you'll get sick!" These physicians demonstrate how this principle can be applied to the art of healing—how we can promote our body's health and stamina through such techniques as meditation, massage (and other types of "laying on of hands"), visualization, yoga exercises, and even joke-telling.

Even Hippocrates knew in 200 B.C. that there was a relationship between emotions and health, when he advised "Let no one persuade you to cure the headache, until he has first given you his soul to be cured. For this is the great error of our day in the treatment of the human body, that physicians separate the soul from the body."

In the meantime, there has been a parallel development in the world of pure medical science that corroborates at the biochemical and neurological levels much of what these holistic doctors believe. This development is the relatively new field of psychoneuroimmunology (PNI), the study of the mechanisms by which psychological and neurological factors affect our immune system.

Age, Immunity, and Age-Immunity

As I stated earlier, the longer we live, the weaker our immune systems become. And this weakness begins distressingly early: just as the incidence of infectious diseases such as pneumonia and influenza rises exponentially after age twenty-five, there are similar statistics for digestive problems, skin rashes, urinary tract infections—the whole list of age-associated infectious diseases. Not only do we run into trouble with our normally "friendly" microbe population as we get older, we also become less efficient at detecting and dealing with new foreign microbes that we bring into our bodies through the air we breathe and the food and water we consume. This is thought to be one of the principal reasons why we are increasingly more likely to develop cancer as we age. A compromised immune system is simply not conducive to a long Youthspan.

The gradual deterioration of the immune system that occurs with age is at least partly the result of a lifetime of chronic exposure to free radicals and that is why the Triple-Your-Youthspan Program emphasizes the use of antioxidants and the avoidance of free-radical-generating toxins in our environment. But you do not have to be elderly to experience a disabled immune system. For decades now, research has shown that the accumulated effect of chronic stress seriously contributes to disabling our immune system regardless of our age. Even in a relatively young person, persistent stress can very quickly produce an "old," ineffective immune system that cannot hold its own against the germs and viruses that regularly set up housekeeping in our bodies. This is basically due to biological changes—particularly hormonal changes—that suppress the ability of the immune system to regulate microbes.

Some convincing evidence for this was revealed recently by the National Institute of Mental Health. In studies of twenty-six forty-year-old women, half of whom were chronically depressed and half not, those with depression had chronically elevated levels of the stress hormones cortisol and the catecholamines. More tellingly, the depressed women had bone densities comparable to seventy-year-old women, while the non-depressed women in the study had normal bone densities for women their age. This was unsurprising, since it is known that chronically elevated levels of stress hormones cause bone reabsorption with the natural outcome of weaker bones and a greater incidence of fractures. Other studies demonstrate that stress and the consequent elevation of stress hormones significantly increase the likelihood of sickness, particularly in women.

Dumb, Short-Term Planning Again

This time it is our stressed-out brain itself that gets us into trouble by reacting to an immediate problem without considering the long-term effects of its response. Our brain signals our adrenal glands to shoot out hormones that help our bodies respond quickly, efficiently, and bravely to some incoming stressor. But over time these very same hormones can wreck our immune system. Stressors can be either physical (say, a sharp change in temperature) or psychological (say, the words, "You're fired!"), the latter being the kind of stressors that we "civilized" humans specialize in. A stressor can be as sudden as a scream or as grindingly drawn out as the drone of traffic outside your bedroom window. There is even growing evidence that a windowless, claustrophobic, fluorescent-lit work cubicle can set up a major stress reaction that we might call the "Dilbert response"—an unperceived reaction that nonetheless does a real number on our nervous system. (Long before psychoneuroimmunology [PNI] came along, the writer Norman Mailer opined that ugly buildings could cause cancer.)

While most physical stressors are introduced to our brain via similar nerves that conduct pain signals from our skin and muscles, most psychological stressors enter our brain through auditory and/ or visual neural pathways that lead to that portion of our brain known as the limbic system. If the limbic system determines that the information it has received is indeed stressful and not, say, a false alarm ("Just kidding, you're not really fired."), it goes into the typical "flight or fight" response: your blood is shunted from your skin (which consequently turns pale) to where it is needed, your muscles; your heart rate increases, pumping extra blood to your internal organs and muscles; glucose (the major blood sugar) is rapidly released from your liver so that it can be used as energy by your muscle cells; your pupils dilate, so that you can see every threat clearly. In short, your brain quickly prepares your body to do one of the two things needed to insure survival—to fight like hell or to run like hell.

Let's take a closer look at the neurochemical sequence that manages this response: the brain's limbic system sends out its "prepare for action" signal to these various body parts via a group of nerves known as the "sympathetic nervous system." Some of these nerves go to the inner portion of our adrenal glands (the adrenal medulla), causing it to release into your blood the hormones called epinephrine (also known as adrenaline) and norepinephrine. And these two compounds mediate the physiological changes of shunting blood from skin to muscle, dilating the pupils, etc.

This is fine for the moment, but when these two hormones linger in our bloodstream trouble begins, and that is exactly what they are wont to do when we are under chronic stress and our bodies are regularly in "flight or fight" mode. Epinephrine and norepinephrine will now curtail the activity of several types of white blood cells that are crucial to our immune system, particularly the white blood cells known as macrophages and lymphocytes, making the body prone to colds and flus and any number of chronic, debilitating infections. Not my idea of a great trade-off, especially since all this stress has a cumulative destructive effect on our immune system as we get older.

There is a second, slower hormonal response of the brain to a stressor through a pathway called the hypothalamo-pituitary-adrenal axis. During long-term stress, the hypothalamus sends a hormone to the pituitary gland, which sends a hormone to the adrenal cortex, which then releases the steroid hormone, cortisol. Once again, the introduction of a hormone into our system has terrific short-term effects, but disastrous long-term effects. Cortisol is fabulous for emergencies: synthetic versions of it are used by physicians to reduce deadly brain swelling, counter perilous allergic reactions, and control dangerous asthma attacks, just to name a few of its powers. But if it remains in our plasma over longer periods of time, it not only seriously compromises our immune system, it may actually permanently damage the hippocampus, that part of our brain that is so important for cataloging our memories.

Dr. Robert Sapolsky, a nationally known neuroscientist working at Stanford University, has published a great deal of animal research which clearly shows that chronic stress is damaging to the hippocampus of animals. In 1996, he published a paper in *Science* that provided new evidence that chronically high levels of stress hormones in humans may be damaging to our hippocampus as well.

There are two basic ways to terminate the biological events that occur during the stress response: either remove the stressor or adapt to it. Removing the stressor may sometimes mean making a significant life change, like quitting a job or moving away from a noisy neighborhood. Adapting to a stressor may sometimes mean what used to be called "grinning and bearing it." And then there is the third solution: don't have the stress response in the first place. This essentially means enhancing your tolerance to stressors, making yourself less reactive to stressors that are not genuine major threats to your well-being. It is primarily this solution that my program subscribes to.

Feedback and Rotary Traffic

Each month, new PNI research adds more evidence that the nervous system and the immune system are profoundly related. Some of these experiments show how maternal separation has a pronounced negative effect on an abandoned child's immune system; others demonstrate how crowding suppresses several aspects of immunity; and still others show how the quality of caregiving to sick patients is reflected in their immune responses. Some of this research shows how depression directly deregulates immune response via the pituitary-adrenal system with the end result of making depressed people much more susceptible to colds and flus.

And then there is the research that shows how traffic flows the other way too, from the immune system back to the nervous system. In one such study, injecting subjects with a substance that stimulated immune cells clearly elevated the subjects' mood. I find this a truly remarkable phenomenon with far-reaching implications. Apparently, communication goes both ways all the time—from body to brain and brain to body. But it is not simply a two-way street, it is more like rotary traffic—a constantly revolving cycle of cause and effect. We know that depression causes our immunological resistance to colds to drop, but it also appears to be true that once the cold takes hold it initiates a hormonal response that causes our depression to deepen . . . and this, in turn, causes our resistance to the cold virus to drop even further. For those of us who are designing strategies for extending Youthspan, such cycles have a profound implication: wherever we are able to intervene on this cycle, we can have an ameliorative effect on both our immune system and our nervous system, on both body and brain.

My Spin on the Youth Cycle

For those of you who are about to embark on the Triple-Your-Youthspan Program, the concept of mind-body rotary traffic has special significance. Primarily, it means that the most dependable way to remain youthful for the longest possible time is by working with both the mind and the body simultaneously with all the means—from the chemical to the spiritual—that are available to us. If meditation makes our nervous system produce more hormones that keep our immune system shipshape and fewer of those that disable it, then by all means we should include meditation in our program. If taking supplements of the hormone DHEA elevates our moods, increases our mental acuity, and causes our nervous systems to produce more immune-stimulating hormones, then we should include it as well. If certain kinds of exercise boost our production of brain endorphins, thereby helping us to think and feel younger and more optimistic, which, in turn, boosts our immune systems, those exercises should also be an option.

But before I get into some general strategies for getting our systems happily spinning in a "Youth Cycle," I have to raise a couple of warning flags about some mind-over-body thinking that is in vogue these days.

The Naturalist's Fallacy

As a holistic-minded scientist, I am delighted by the current popular rediscovery of the role mind and mood play in fighting disease and promoting good health. The books of Dr. Bernie Siegal and Dr. Andrew Weil have opened up doctors and patients alike to the health-promoting powers of meditation, touch, visualization, general stress reduction, and prayer. As we will see, many of these techniques and practices work synergistically with the drug and supplement aspects of my program. Besides offering alternative and supplementary therapies for a wide range of diseases, this new awareness of the mind's capacity to heal has proved to be a powerful antidote to the general coldness and impersonality of late twentieth-century medicine.

One doctor I know told me that after reading one of Dr. Siegal's books he realized that up to that point he had only had direct physical contact with his patients when absolutely necessary.

"It was tantamount to treating them like pariahs, to saying to them, 'You're so diseased I cannot even stand to touch you,' " he told me. "So now when I take a patient's blood pressure or test his reflexes, I pause to pat his back or knead his shoulders. And, by God, I can see that it really does help them get better. If that's 'healing hands,' I'm all for it."

Yet in righting an imbalance in the way modern medicine is practiced, some mind-over-body healers have created a few serious problems of their own. One of these is to put a patient in the position of blaming herself for a disease she may contract, the medical variation of blaming the victim. I have seen this as a hospice volunteer. Sometimes a patient with a terminal disease will be referred to us because, in the words of their physicians, "They failed their treatment." And perhaps more tragically, as a patient is only referred to us if he or she is believed to have fewer than six months to live, some hospice patients actually begin to feel guilty if they do not die within their allotted six months.

I have also experienced this unhappy phenomenon with a friend of mine who was dying from an inoperable brain tumor. A well-meaning neighbor of this woman visited her frequently, always bringing along visualization tapes to help her "fight the cancer with her mind." One of these tapes asserted unequivocally that the chief cause of cancer was "negative thinking," and my weakened friend started to blame herself for her fatal disease, thrusting her into even deeper despair. To me, this is a wrong-headed and unconscionable burden to put on any person suffering from ill health.

There is another error that many mind-over-body healers commit in the name of natural purity, one that is particularly relevant to the Triple-Your-Youthspan Program. And that is the mistake of believing that because a certain state of mind has the clear effect of enhancing your health, the only legitimate way to achieve this state of mind is through psychological or spiritual means—that is, through nonchemical means like yoga, meditation, massage, prayer, or talk therapy. For these holistic purists, evidence that relieving depression enhances resistance to common cold viruses implies that the mind is supreme, so the mind should be dealt with solely and directly to set this neuroimmune sequence in action. To them, dealing with the mind directly through its brain chemistry would somehow be "cheating" or not showing the mind proper respect. And so they disdain trying to counter the virus-friendly depression via chemical means, say with a naturally occurring amino acid like L-tryptophan, a synthetic hormone supplement like DHEA, a drug like Prozac, or even a "natural" herb like St. John's wort, all of which have been shown to combat depression.

Not long ago, I debated this very question with a friend who is deeply committed to holistic medicine. I had come across some findings that clinically depressed people who began taking St. John's wort actually caught fewer colds than before taking the drug. This evidence, although anecdotal, suggested that relieving depression through chemical means had the same (or even possibly stronger) effect on the immune system as relieving the depression through mental or spiritual means, like yoga or psychotherapy. But my holistic friend was unimpressed. "It's not a good idea to interrupt the mind-body cycle artificially," he argued. "You aren't really healing the person that way, you are just temporarily relieving the symptoms."

But if "artificially" interrupting the cycle sets that cycle spinning up and away from both present and future depression and infections, I am all for it. I am only interested in pure results (better health), not in the so-called purity of the means to those results.

Some Late-Night Thoughts on Synergy

I say this because I am an inveterate pragmatist: if something works and is affordable but not harmful, I am for it. And that is not simply because I believe in a "shotgun" approach to extending Youthspan—that is, covering as many contingencies as possible by using all strategies that have proven efficacious—but because it turns out that there is genuine synergy to these various strategies. These combined strategies have more than a cumulative (additive) effect; they actually appear to have a multiplying effect on each other.

Let's extend the above example. If an individual is in general prone to both colds and depression and takes substantial daily doses of immune-enhancing vitamins, minerals, and hormones to guard against the former, and doses of St. John's wort to guard against the latter, he will probably enjoy the benefits of this multiplying effect: the vitamins, minerals, and hormones will strengthen his immune system, which, in turn, will enhance his resistance to depression; the St. John's wort will enhance his resistance to depression, which, in turn, will strengthen his immune system. And it appears that the net effect of taking both the supplements and the St. John's wort will be mind-body rotary traffic spiraling upward to ever stronger resistance to germs and depression, each supplement enhancing the effect of the other. Now let's say we add to this mix a regular program of meditation that has the effect of further enhancing one's tolerance to stressors, and to that we add other hormone supplements that are known to directly enhance mood. Each additional element has the potential to affect the others—and very quickly the multiplication effect gets awfully heady.

Thinking Young as a Self-Fulfilling Biological Fantasy

Some of the directed meditations and fantasy mind exercises that are part of my program will undoubtedly strike some readers as pretty silly stuff—but I haven't gone soft in the head. I'm just exceedingly practical. It seems that the old adage, "Thinking young helps you feel young" has a testable biological correlative: people who regularly "delude" themselves into believing that they are younger than their actual age are probably going to have stronger immune systems and a higher tolerance for stressors than people who resign themselves to "growing old." That is because seeing yourself as losing your youth is itself stressful and depressing, with a negative effect on the immune system.

Examples of this can be seen in sick people. A 1988 study looked at behavioral training over one year in cancer patients (who are very often stressed out and depressed), using guided imagery or progressive muscle relaxation. This training resulted in significant improvements in several immune parameters, such as T-lymphocyte function, the activity of natural killer cells, and the production of interleuken 2 by lymphocytes. In addition, in a 1989 study, breast cancer patients who met weekly in psychological support groups lived about twice as long as similar patients receiving no such support. Physicians and scientists had long known that people with a brighter outlook on life lived longer and healthier lives, but now they were finally seeing some of the physiological reasons for this.

One final thought here about "rotary traffic": We all have a tendency (myself included) to focus on the ways in which a tranquil, positive mind can bestow healthy and healing benefits on the body. But an attenuated Youthspan calls for a positive attitude in general, a pervasive optimism, a *joie de vivre*. One's Youthspan is, by its very nature, a period of life that is relatively free of melancholy and pessimism. And so when we allow ourselves to embrace life and new experiences, that too strengthens our bodies and minds, and so enables us to extend our Youthspan.

The oncologist and DHEA advocate Dr. William Regelson once told me that he had devised his own method for gauging depression. He said, "When I am speaking to an audience, I ask them 'If I could give you another thirty years of healthy life by using DHEA and other supplements, would you take it?' Those people who say no are definitely clinically depressed."

CHAPTER FIVE

The Charts

*I*f you want to stay thirty, it is best to begin this program at thirty or even earlier, then add elements to it at forty and fifty. For example, hormone replacement enters the program mostly at around age fifty when natural production of testosterone in men, estrogen in women, and DHEA and growth hormone in both men and women begin to get critically low, so as to produce age-related symptoms. Some as-needed elements of the program, like nootropics, may be appropriate as early as age thirty. And, of course, in this nation of couch potatoes and fast-food addicts, it is never too early to begin a simple routine of physical exercise and a calorie-modified, saturated fat-, cholesterol-, and sodium-restricted diet.

What follows are my dosage charts for twenty and over, thirty and over, forty and over, and fifty and over. Except for certain as-needed supplements, the program is cumulative: at thirty, you take everything you did at twenty, plus some new additions; at forty, you take everything you did at thirty, plus other new additions, etc. Some elements of the program can only be taken in the United States at this time by prescription; and some of the hormone supplements should only be taken under the supervision of a physician who monitors their effects.

In Part IV, you will find a detailed description of each element of the program, including what forms of certain supplements are most effective, the recommended way to calculate certain body weight-specific dosages, how to space out dosages, specific brain exercises and antistress techniques, and diet and physical exercise guidelines. But if Part IV is the meat and potatoes of my program, the charts that follow are the recipes— you will undoubtedly find yourself referring back to them on a regular basis once you are committed to extending your Youthspan.

AGE 20 AND OVER

Youth Enhancer	Dosage	Precautions
Relaxation Techniques	Daily Meditation, 15+ minutes	None
Physical Exercise	Aerobic, 3 times a week, 20 minutes	Physical examination for high blood pressure and heart disease.
Diet	Calorie and Saturated Fat Restrictions	Do not consume fewer calories than you expend daily.
Nootropics	As needed at first signs of cognitive/memory loss; see chart below	(see chart below)

Nootropics can be taken individually or in combination. As effects vary greatly from individual to individual, I recommend starting with one, then adding others one at a time as desired, waiting a few weeks between each addition to gauge its effect. I have listed them below in the order I suggest you take them; that is, start with Gingko biloba, then add acetyl-L-carnitine, etc.

Nootropics

Nootropic	Indication	Daily Dosage	Precaution
Gingko Biloba	Memory loss	120 milligrams divided in 3 equal doses	None
Acetyl-L-Carnitine (ALC)	General cognitive loss	500–2000 milligrams/day; divided in 3 equal doses	Decrease dosage if dizziness, stomach distress, restlessness, or hyperactivity occurs.

Nootropics (cont.)

Hydergine *[need prescription from Doctor (U.S.A.) use with piracetam]*	Declining alertness	3 milligrams/day in 3 equal doses *[need 3 x day]*	Halve dosage if nausea, gastric distress, or headache occurs.
Phosphatidylserine	General cognitive loss	300 milligrams/day in 3 equal doses	None
Piracetam *[can't buy in the USA]*	General cognitive loss	2400–4800 milligrams divided into 3 doses.	None
Centrophenoxine (CPH) *[can't buy in USA]*	Loss of alertness	1000 milligrams in 2 equal doses	None

AGE 30 AND OVER

Youth Enhancer	Daily Dosage	Precautions
Vitamin & Mineral Antioxidants		
Beta Carotene	15 to 20 milligrams every other day	If skin turns yellow/orange reduce dosage
Mixed Carotenoids	50 to 100 milligrams every other day	None
Vitamin E	400 IUs	Consult your physician if you are using blood-thining medications.
Vitamin C	500 milligrams	None
Selenium	200 micrograms every other day	Signs of selenium poisoning (rare): muscle twitching, lethargy, hair loss, abdominal cramps, white streaking in nails, or nails falling out.
Nonvitamin & Mineral Antioxidants		
Coenzyme Q-10	50–100 milligrams	None
Glutathione	100–200 milligrams	None
N-acetyl-L cysteine (NAC)	100–200 milligrams	None
Alpha Lipoic Acid (ALA)	100–200 milligrams	None
Pycnogenol or Grape seed	By body weight, see details in "Mega-Chicken Soup"	None

AGE 30 AND OVER (cont.)

Other Essential Vitamins and Minerals

Folic Acid	1–2 milligrams	If you have a vitamin B12 deficiency or are receiving drugs for seizures or an existing cancer, consult your physician before taking folic acid supplements.
Zinc	30 milligrams	If irritates stomach, halve dosage.

Essential Fatty Acids

Mixed Omega-3	One gram (1000 milligrams)	None

Antiinflammatories

Aspirin	325 milligrams (one adult tablet every other day)	Can cause ulcers and internal bleeding in greater amounts.

AGE 40 AND OVER

Youth Enhancer	Daily Dosage	Precautions
Hormone Replacement: Melatonin	.5 milligrams–10 milligrams half hour before retiring; start with lowest amount, build by .5-milligram doses to desired amount	Causes drowsiness—do not take during day or before driving; adjust dose so you are not drowsy day after.
Hormone Replacement: DHEA	Start at 25 milligrams, add by 25-milligram increments	Can elevate PSA; have PSA tested and digital prostate exam before starting; ideally, have blood plasma DHEA and androgens assayed before starting.
Hormone Replacement: Estrogen	Consult physician at onset of menopause	Can elevate risk for certain cancers; see details, consult physician.

AGE 40 AND OVER (cont.)

Physical Exercises: Anaerobic	20–30 minutes 3 times per week	Can cause muscle strain—build weights gradually; best under supervision.
Brain Exercises	15 minutes daily of cognitive functions you are not regularly using; see details	None

AGE 50 AND OVER

Youth Enhancer	Daily Dosage	Precautions
Hormone Replacement: Testosterone	Consult physician	Can elevate PSA; have PSA tested and digital prostate exam before starting; have plasma free testosterone assayed before starting.
Hormone Replacement: Growth Hormone	Consult physician	Can induce carpal tunnel syndrome and/or glucose intolerance—if so, decrease or discontinue dosage; have plasma insulin-like growth factors assayed, as well as a GH-provocation test before starting.
Relaxation Techniques: Visualization Exercises	10–15 minutes daily	None

What the Program Is, How It Works,
and How to Do It

*I*n the following sections, we get down to the details of my program, delineating the supplements, mental and physical exercises, antistress techniques, and dietary guidelines that work together to promote a long and healthy Youthspan.

In the charts above, the program was broken down according to the optimal age when each aspect of it should be phased in. Now, it is broken down by elements of Youthspan: brain functions (The Smarts), immune system (Mega-Chicken Soup), strength and vitality (Flab Into Muscle and Sloth Into Energy), mood and sexuality (Feeling Young and Sexy), and physical appearance (Hey, Good-Looking).

In each of these sections, I describe the basic tools that work for it, but I should say at the outset that virtually all of the tools in this program contribute to more than one element of Youthspan and most of them work synergistically with one another. For this reason, there is a certain amount of arbitrariness to where each tool is described; for example, I discuss antioxidants in Mega-Chicken Soup, but I could have just as reasonably discussed them under The Smarts because antioxidants are critical in keeping brain cells alive and active. Nonetheless, by the end of this book every Youthspan Tool—what it is, how it works, and how to use it—is thoroughly explored.

One of my Over-Thirty Basketball League buddies says that you know you are getting older when you tell more jokes that take place in doctors' offices than in bedrooms. Well, the aging jokes I hear (and tell) most frequently are about short-term memory loss. Most of us experience cognitive deficit before we experience any other age-related deficits, and invariably this fills us with a nervous foreboding. The main reason for this is that we tend to see these early minor lapses of memory as previews of the dementia that must be on its way. When we forget where we parked the car in the railway station lot, we become convinced that Alzheimer's disease is waiting for us right around the corner.

Chances are that your current minor lapses are unrelated to your proclivity to Alzheimer's disease in later years. Nonetheless, I am happy to report that many of the precautions and therapies that you can use to keep from having these little lapses may also lessen your likelihood of contracting Alzheimer's and other dementias later on.

Much of what we call forgetting a fact, image, or incident actually means that we never paid sufficient attention to that fact, image, or incident in the first place and so it did not make a sufficient impression on us to be remembered. Thus, if a supplement or brain exercise improves our ability to actively focus on what is going on around us or what we are reading, we will be more likely to store it away for later use.

Another critical area of cognition that concerns us is what cognitive psychologists call "word retrieval," the ability to instantly pull out the right word when you want to use it. The decline of this faculty is one of the most dreaded hallmarks of a waning Youthspan.

Intelligence encompasses many functions, from general cognitive power to the ability to process new information and make logical decisions based on this information. It is foresight, verbal recall, comprehension of new information, abstraction, and competent decision-making, to name just a few functions. The list of cognitive functions that can be enhanced by estrogen, testosterone, and DHEA hormone-replacement therapy (mostly after age fifty), nootropics, and antioxidants, as well as brain exercises and relaxation techniques, goes on and on: improved abstract reasoning and problem-solving, a higher degree of reading comprehension—even a quicker

DOES STRESS MAKE YOU SLOW-WITTED?
OR, DOES A SLOW BRAIN STRESS YOU OUT?

If you have a job and/or lifestyle that constantly puts multiple demands on your attention, as you reach middle age you may literally find yourself being driven to distraction; the phone rings just as someone steps into your office and you feel a flush of anxiety that induces you to do something dumb or inappropriate like greeting your caller by the wrong name or momentarily forgetting the reason you asked your office visitor to meet with you. If repeated often enough, the long-term consequences of this kind of fumble will be loss of confidence and lowered self-esteem. In short, this is the kind of thing that makes you feel very old.

Is stress the cause of this kind of blunder, or is the stress a result of the anxiety caused by foggy responses? The answer, of course, is that both are true: it's rotary-traffic time again. And so a reasonable approach to the problem would be to find ways to both lower stress and to increase cognitive function.

DHEA or estrogen-replacement therapy might very well be in order; both can increase mental energy and endurance while calming nerves. Likewise, the drug Piracetam and the compound phosphatidylserine could increase the mental agility needed to juggle tasks. Stress reduction alone would be important: physical exercise and a relaxation technique like transcendental meditation could make a substantial difference here.

wit. How, you may wonder, can these various techniques target these disparate mental functions?

The answer lies more in the miraculous talents of the brain than in the various therapies that revive and empower the brain. Healthy brains are capable of all these functions; the drugs and exercises merely keep them healthy and youthful enough to perform them. To be sure, different specific therapies appear to have greater impact on certain functions than others (when I discuss dosage, I will address these differences accordingly). For example, many users associate Hydergine with a heightened ability to concentrate and to

A LOSS FOR WORDS

Have you ever been in full swing making a presentation at work and suddenly found yourself stumbling, "Uh, er, the, uh . . . what's it called? You know what I mean."

A result of this kind of slip is a kind of nervousness that makes it increasingly difficult for you to find the right word as you go on, compounding the problem. Not good for your career. Or for your mental health.

A regime of phosphatidylserine and Ginkgo biloba could make a major difference in your life. In addition, a course of brain exercises—particular memory exercises—to increase synaptic plasticity could pay off in better word retrieval.

memory

keep track of details. And brain exercises that focus on memory function tend to enhance that function more than others. But in general, of course, improving one cognitive function almost always results in improving all other cognitive functions.

LOSING IT?

Are you concerned that someone you know may have more than normal age-associated cognitive loss? One way to screen for a more serious problem that requires medical intervention is to do a brief mental screening exam. You can do this by going to http://www.alz.uci.edu/screen2.html on the Internet, where you will find a list of short dementia-screening tests provided by the Institute for Brain Aging at the University of California, Irvine, that you can actually use online. Although there are several listed, I suggest clicking on the Mini Mental State Exam, which was designed by Dr. Marshall Folstein, a psychiatrist at Boston University. You can administer this exam and score it right on your computer. You then submit it for evaluation to the Institute for Brain Aging right over the Internet.

Because of the complexity of the brain as well as the varying definitions of what intelligence is, the use of smart drugs is not an exact science. But as long as these compounds that enhance some components of what we call intelligence are proven without a doubt to be safe, and are effective in many people, we clearly should vigorously pursue further testing of these compounds. This has been occurring in Europe for many years, and I believe smart drugs will become a big market here as well; pharmaceutical companies know that Americans put a high value on intellectual power.

The subjective results of the Triple-Your-Youthspan Program are sometimes more spectacular than the objective results, and the outcomes in brain function are certainly no exception. But in the long run, the objective results have as much, if not more, to do with your lengthened Youthspan. You may not have any subjective indication that your brain is doing a better job of dealing with free radicals or generating less oxidative stress, but the blood markers that reveal these results mean that your chances of keeping your brain young and healthy have been markedly improved.

SECURITY IN NUMBERS

When it comes to age-related dementia, one of our greatest fears is fear itself. Even if we are doing everything in our power to avoid this dreaded disease—taking the antioxidants and hormones that guard against free radical damage to our neurons—we may still live in terror of brain deterioration. That is one good reason why you should regularly get a blood assay to determine the antioxidant capacity of your blood, as well as a test for urinary levels of markers of oxidative stress. If these numbers confirm that your blood is resistant to oxidation, it means your brain is probably more resistant to the ravages of age-related degeneration as well, so you can give your fear a well-deserved rest. See Genox Corporation under "Diagnostic Testing Sites" in the Resources section at the back of the book for information on these tests.

CHAPTER SIX

Smart Tools I: Smart Drugs and Nutrients

*N*ootropics (Greek for "mind-turning") are an innovative class of synthetic and naturally occurring compounds that actually boost the capacity of the "normal" brain in a wide range of ways. They are compounds that can produce a subjective effect in our thinking quite quickly—for minutes to days. This can be experienced in a heightened ability to take an exam, a greater facility at recalling words or events, a better ability to concentrate or to perform any of the other tasks that we associate with intelligence.

The effects of these smart drugs contrast with the effects of most of the other substances in my program, which do not immediately produce any subjective effects or change in cognitive function, but rather work to protect the brain and body from damage over the years, minimizing our chances of losing cognitive functions, or getting some form of dementia or other serious age-related disease in our sixth or seventh decade.

The use of smart drugs is controversial. Some have called them drugs in search of a disease, because they do not compensate for a cognitive loss so much as they enhance normal cognitive abilities. Remember, the FDA and the conventional medical community do not condone the use of drugs for something that they do not deem a clinical disease; in other words, if you feel you have lost your cognitive edge, but this loss is not considered by a neurologist to be part of a recognized affliction, your condition is deemed normal and nothing will be done for you. And if you do not feel that you have undergone any cognitive loss, but are nonetheless eager to see if your mind can operate at a higher level through the use of a safe, nontoxic synthetic or naturally occurring substance, the FDA and your conventional doctor will strongly advise against it.

Why, you may ask, do they have such a problem with cognitive enhancement while they approve one drug and surgery after another for beauty enhancement? Is baldness a disease? Are face lifts or breast implants greater requirements for a healthy, satisfying life than an increased memory?

For me, the sine qua non of a long and healthy Youthspan is a quick and retentive mind. Therefore, I have made nootropics an important option in the Triple-Your-Youthspan Program for anyone with even an inkling of memory-retention problems.

Naturally Occurring Nootropics

Several naturally occurring, nonprescription compounds have shown promise as cognitive function enhancers, although their efficacy seems to vary considerably from person to person. All of the ones that I suggest here are safe.

Gingko Biloba

WHAT IT IS AND HOW IT WORKS

Gingko biloba is an extract of the leaf of the Gingko biloba tree, which grows in many places in Europe, and is one of the oldest trees known to exist today. Physicians in Europe write over one million prescriptions a year for Gingko biloba extract, particularly for peripheral vascular disease. It is now well established that Gingko biloba increases blood flow to the brain and so, predictably, has been shown to be particularly effective in alleviating memory disorders in the elderly that are related to a reduced blood flow to their brains. In fact, several studies show that people suffering from cerebral insufficiency (lack of adequate blood flow to the brain) are able to perform significantly better on tests of short-term memory and rates of learning after taking Gingko biloba extracts for only six to twenty-four weeks. In one double-blind, placebo-controlled study, a group of patients over fifty who showed mild to moderate memory impairment took an oral dose of a standardized Gingko biloba extract three times a day. At the end of twelve to twenty-four weeks, a series of cognitive tests was administered and only those patients taking the Gingko biloba extract showed significant improvement in cognitive function.

Furthermore, as noted in a 1997 study published in the *Journal of the American Medical Association,* forty milligrams of Gingko biloba taken three times daily with meals significantly improved many cognitive parameters in patients with Alzheimer's Disease and multi-infarct dementia.

Many other examples of memory enhancement are found in the literature. People with cerebral-organic syndrome (which causes dizziness, and memory and concentration loss) have been shown to improve dramatically after four and eight weeks of daily supplements of Gingko biloba extract. But perhaps most tellingly, healthy people with no detectable clinical cognitive problems have been shown to improve in choice-reaction times, subjective rating scales, and memory-scanning tests after taking Gingko biloba extract.

Gingko biloba is also a proven treatment for some age-related mood disorders, in particular depression. It has been shown that individuals with cerebral insufficiency often suffer from depression; and in a clinical trial involving sixty patients with both cerebral insufficiency and depressive mood, 160 milligrams of Gingko biloba extract daily significantly improved symptoms of both problems.

Gingko biloba (60 milligrams daily) has also been found to effectively increase blood flow to the penis in patients with erectile dysfunction, when used for six to eight weeks or more.

DOSAGE*

Although primarily known as a nootropic, Gingko biloba happily doubles as a potent antioxidant because of its flavonoid glycosides, so I do not hesitate to recommend it to everyone in the program.

---

*Unless otherwise indicated, dosages apply to both men and women of all body weights.

But in general, because of its expense and because there are other even more effective antioxidant supplements available, I only recommend its use to people who feel they have started to suffer some small cognitive loss, especially in short-term memory, or to people who simply believe their lives would be significantly improved by greater mental acuity. Used alone or in combination with other nootropics, it can enhance cognition effectively and rather rapidly.

Most Gingko biloba sold in the U.S. is in a standardized 50:1 extract (with each tablet containing 24 percent flavonoid glycosides and 6 percent terpenes). You can buy the tablets with varying milligrams of Gingko biloba extract. It has been shown that as little as 150 milligrams daily of this extract (one fifty-milligram tablet taken three times a day) significantly improves various types of memory. Again, you are best off being your own doctor here, *staring with the 150-milligram dose for four weeks and working the dose upward if there is insufficient improvement.* I would not recommend more than 600 milligrams daily.

One effective way for you to calculate the optimum dosage of Gingko biloba (or for other nootropics or combinations of nootropics) is to set up a simple baseline for yourself of a few critical cognitive functions. I recommend memorizing random number strings to test your short-term memory and playing one of the many eye-hand-reflex video games like Tetris or Mario Brothers to test your reaction time. Test yourself again after four weeks of taking 150 milligrams of Gingko biloba daily. If you do not perform any better, you will want to up your dosage to 200 or 250 milligrams a day, and test yourself a third time after another four weeks. If in the first test you do perform better, you may still want to increase your dosage for another four-week period to determine if you can improve your cognitive functions even more.

If you are taking Gingko biloba to relieve depression, I recommend starting at around *160 milligrams daily* and increasing by increments of fifty milligrams until your mood is effectively elevated.

A bonus: tinnitus, or ringing in the ears, is thought to affect some fifty million Americans, the majority of them middle-aged or older. Generally if you have this problem, your doctor will tell you to live with it, because he will say there are no known treatments for it (although some types can be treated). However, some recent clinical trials show that Gingko biloba extract is an effective treatment for this disorder in doses of *150 to 200 milligrams daily,* taken in three divided doses.

Acetyl-L-Carnitine

WHAT IT IS AND HOW IT WORKS

Acetyl-L-carnitine (ALC) is a synthetic, acetylated version of the naturally occurring nitrogenous substance L-carnitine. This is a substance that enhances oxidative phosphorylation (ATP production in the mitochondria) by supplying the mitochondria with certain fatty acids it needs. Taking oral L-carnitine does not greatly increase the supply of carnitine to the brain cells (although it does to nonbrain cells) since it does not readily cross the blood-brain barrier; but by sticking an acetyl group on the L-carnitine molecule and forming ALC, we can cross this barrier and thus supply the brain with extra L-carnitine.

Animal studies have shown ALC prevents age-related lipid peroxidation of brain cells and age-associated reduction in nerve growth factor, a critical substance for maintaining normal functioning in the mammalian brain. Other studies show that ALC shields the brain from age-induced damage, including protecting NMDA receptors in the hippocampus against damage by free radicals.

Dozens of clinical trials, mostly in Europe, have been conducted with ALC to measure its effects on cognitive functions. For example, a 1992 study in Italy found that when seventeen healthy young people were given ALC or a placebo for thirty days, and were tested before and after for attention levels, reflexes, and hand-eye coordination, reflex speed was significantly improved, and errors and task completion time significantly reduced in those using ALC.

People with senile dementia and in the early stages of Alzheimer's disease also experience improvements in cognitive functions after administration of oral ALC. One example of this is a 1992 study out of the Department of Nutrition at Georgia State University which found that people with Alzheimer's disease who received 2,000 milligrams of ALC each day for a year experienced a significant reduction in the progress of their disease compared to those not taking ALC supplements.

DOSAGE

Acetyl-L-carnitine (ALC) is in a league of its own both as a nootropic compound and as a neuroprotector. The dosages used in the clinical trials of humans which support the use of ALC for improvement of cognitive functioning range from 500 to 2,000 milligrams per day. The reason for these relatively high dosages is to ensure that the ALC maintains its "acetyl" group that makes it more fat soluble, thus allowing it to leave the bloodstream and enter into the brain.

Almost all the ALC capsules you can order come in either 250- or 500-milligram capsules. Whichever dose of ALC you select to start with should be split up into three separate doses throughout the day, and administered with food each time. In other words, should you choose to take 1,500 milligrams daily (a popular dosage), you should take *500 milligrams three times a day,* with food. This seems to be a very safe dosage; the only side effects that on rare occasions have been reported are vertigo (dizziness), abdominal discomfort, restlessness, and hyperactivity. If you experience any of these symptom using ALC, cut back your dosage until the symptoms disappear.

Because it has been proven so effective for so many people, ALC is one of the most expensive substances that are discussed in this book, costing around fifty to sixty dollars a month to use at dosages that are effective. I personally hope that this important and effective substance can be supplied at a more reasonable cost in the near future.

Hydergine

WHAT IT IS AND HOW IT WORKS

Hydergine is an extract of ergot, a fungus that grows on some plants. It was one of the first natural compounds to be tried in the treatment of Alzheimer's disease and has shown benefits in the treatment of several kinds of senile dementias. A recent analysis of several clinical trials concluded that overall, ergot mesylates like Hydergine were more effective than placebo in these studies. However, the effect in patients with possible Alzheimer's dementia was modest at best.

Hydergine has been widely used for the therapy of cerebral

vascular disease in humans; it prevents platelets from clotting abnormally and blocking our arteries, including those that supply our hearts and brains with blood, thus reducing the incidence of strokes and heart attacks.

Only in the past fifteen years have its "smart" properties been studied in people who do not have existing dementia. It apparently enhances cognition by providing some protective effect on the brain in people who are subjected to low levels of oxygen there (which often occurs in atherosclerosis), and it can increase the blood flow to the brain, possibly by dilating cerebral blood vessels.

Also, studies done on old rats suggest that Hydergine can actually enhance synaptic plasticity by acting like neural growth factors, the small proteins in the brain that cause certain parts of neurons to "sprout."

DOSAGE

For increasing alertness and cognition, the effective dose of Hydergine is *three milligrams per day, split into three separate doses.* (In clinical trials of people *with dementia,* the benefits of Hydergine were most pronounced in doses of *more than four milligrams daily, divided into three separate doses* throughout the day.) Unlike many other cognitive-enhancing substances, this one can take up to three or four weeks before producing noticeable effects. If you experience nausea, gastric disturbances, or headache when you start using this nootropic, cut the dose in half. If any of these symptoms persist, try a different "smart" drug.

Hydergine can be obtained with a physician's prescription in the United States. If you do not have (or cannot find) a doctor to prescribe it for you, it can be purchased over the counter in Mexico or by mail order from some of the sources listed in Appendix A. Many people believe that Hydergine is most effective when used in conjunction with Piracetam.

Phosphatidylserine

WHAT IT IS AND HOW IT WORKS

Phosphatidylserine (PPS) is a naturally occurring substance that is essential to all cell membranes, but is found in particularly high concentrations in the cell membranes of the brain. Clinical studies have shown that PPS works by supporting certain brain functions that decline with age, possibly by enhancing neurotransmission by neurons and stabilizing neuronal cell membranes. Until recently, PPS was available only from animal sources (their brains), and was found in trace amounts in commercial lecithin, but a plant source of PPS has now been found.

Several studies in older humans have shown that PPS can produce significant improvement in a number of cognitive parameters including attention, concentration, short-term memory, and new memory acquisition. In addition, PPS seems to enhance cognitive functions in young people.

One recent experiment used an electroencephalogram (EEG) to measure brain electrical activity in eight men ages twenty-one to twenty-eight. Baseline EEGs were done, and when PPS was given, it boosted their alpha waves by 15 to 20 percent. Alpha waves are highly indicative of learning/memory activity in the brain; they are often found to be lower in the elderly.

As we have seen, cognitive function and mood are intimately related in people as they age: loss of memory invariably leads to depression; and depression has a pronounced negative effect on all cognitive functions. So it is no surprise that when PPS has been administered to elderly people suffering from depression, their depression has improved significantly.

DOSAGE

The oral dosage of phosphatidylserine (PPS) that has been shown in clinical trials to effectively and safely improve a number of cognitive parameters ranged from 200 to 300 milligrams daily. Most studies used *300 milligrams, given in three, 100-milligram doses throughout the day.* PPS is not abundant in the human diet and we can synthesize it to some extent, but the amounts we synthesize do not appear to be sufficient for maximal cognitive functioning. No serious side effects have been reported at the 300-milligram daily dose.

Synthetic Nootropics

Synthetic nootropics represent a group of compounds that were developed over thirty years ago in Belgium for the treatment of memory loss in patients with various types of dementia. The best known of these is Piracetam (also known as Nootropil), from which many of the other nootropics have been designed, including oxiracetam, pramiracetam, etiracetam, and aniracetam. Synthetic nootropics have been used for decades by millions of people throughout the world with an extremely good safety record; nonetheless, Piracetam is one of the smart drugs that the FDA does not allow to be sold in this country.

Piracetam

WHAT IT IS AND HOW IT WORKS

To this day, there is no general agreement on the mechanism of action of Piracetam and its derivatives. Some studies have suggested that they enhance the activity of the cholinergic system in the brain—a part of the brain that uses the neurotransmitter acetylcholine for memory and learning functions. Neuroscientists have known for years that acetylcholine is a particularly important neurotransmitter involved in the process of storing memories in the mammalian brain, particularly long-term memory storage in the hippocampus. For example, in animal studies, drugs that block the effects of acetylcholine cause severe memory problems. When Piracetam is given along with these acetylcholine-blocking drugs, the loss in memory is often either reversed or greatly alleviated.

Another thing that Piracetam and Piracetam-like drugs seem to do quite well is protect against the disruption of the acquisition of long-term memories. Scientists can erase memories in short-term storage in animals by giving them electroconvulsive stimulation of the brain; when Piracetam and its analogues are given before the electrical stimulation, they effectively guard against this loss of short-term memory, although how they do this is not known.

DOSAGE

Piracetam is usually supplied in 400- and 800-milligram tablets. Most people use a dose of from *2,400 to 4,800 milligrams daily, divided into three doses.* However, it is fairly common for people first using Piracetam to only experience subjective cognitive effects at doses of between 6,000 to 8,000 milligrams daily, in three divided doses. Once a subjective effect is noticed, I advise cutting the dose back down to 2,400 to 4,800 milligrams, in three divided doses daily.

Because users of Piracetam claim that it works synergistically with Centrophenoxine and Hydergine, if you are taking either of these other drugs, you may be able to increase your level of cognitive functioning with smaller doses of each drug in combination, rather than with any one of these substances individually.

Although used throughout Europe for years with an outstanding safety record, Piracetam is not sold in the U.S. It can be bought without a prescription in Mexico, or ordered from some of the companies listed in Appendix A.

Centrophenoxine

WHAT IT IS AND HOW IT WORKS

Centrophenoxine (CPH), also known as meclofenoxate (trade name Lucidril), has been around in Europe for some time, where doctors use it to treat several types of memory disorders. (It has not been approved for use in the U.S.) Chemically, this drug is a combination of p-chlorophenoxyacetic acid and a substance known as dimethylaminoethanol (DMAE), a compound which is normally found in small quantities in our brain.

Apparently, CPH works by preventing accumulation of lipofuscin in the brain—lipofuscin can decrease the electrical activity of the hippocampus, an area of the brain you now know is critical to cognitive functioning. In fact, a recent study suggests that CPH may play a significant role in slowing down brain aging due to its ability to prevent lipofuscin formation. Other studies have shown CPH to affect the important acetylcholine neurotransmitter system in the hippocampus.

CPH has also been shown to affect the membrane fluidity of brain cells, which is very important in allowing the cells to communicate with their surrounding environment. Furthermore, it can block the action of the enzyme monoamine oxidase (MOA) in the brain, which means it probably produces effects similar to some antidepressants. Therefore, do not use this compound if you are currently using any MAO inhibitor drug.

Finally, CPH may not only benefit cognition in the short run, but may also benefit your brain in the long run since CPH has been shown to be a potent scavenger of hydroxyl free radicals. CPH is currently the smart drug of choice for people who believe that you do not have to begin experiencing cognitive loss to start nurturing your cognitive functions.

DOSAGE

For increased alertness and cognitive functioning, start with a dosage of CPH of *1,000 milligrams (500 milligrams in the morning, 500 milligrams with supper)*. If you are taking a dose effective for you, you will notice a change in alertness within minutes. If you do not have this experience, double the dose until you feel an effect, though not more than 4,000 milligrams daily.

Many people believe that CPH works synergistically with Piracetam and Hydergine, so you may be able to take lesser amounts of combinations of these substances than if you were taking any one of them alone.

Like other supplements I recommend that cannot be bought in this country, CPH can be bought over the counter in Mexico or can be ordered from the companies listed in the Resources section under Smart Drug Information or under Domestic Supplement Sources.

A Final Thought

It is difficult for people to objectively determine whether or not they have actually experienced an increase of cognitive function after they have used a "smart drug" for a period of time. Although I suggested some basic ways to do this in the section on Gingko biloba, the most effective way would be to undergo a battery of established neuropsychological tests before using any of these substances, and then again after using one of these compunds for a period of time.

This is not practical or affordable for most people; however, one method that can now be used is a relatively new software program called ThinkFast, available from Cognitive Diagnostics (see Resources) for approximately fifty dollars. In just five to ten minutes, ThinkFast can measure your reaction time, perceptual threshold, attention span, and working memory, among other things.

CHAPTER SEVEN

Smart Tools II: Brain Exercises

What They Are and How They Work

When it comes to brain cells, our first order of business is slowing their rate of death—hence the importance of anti-oxidants. But new evidence suggests another important way we can keep our brain functioning at a high level as we age—by exercising it! The adage "use it or lose it" seems to apply to our brain as much as to our other "muscles." And this, of course, is because of "synaptic plasticity," our ability to remodel synapses by inputting information to our brains.

Different types of brain exercises appear to promote different areas of synaptic plasticity. And exactly what does what is fairly logical and straightforward: memory exercises seem to promote a greater memory reserve; problem-solving exercises seem to promote a greater problem-solving reserve; abstract reasoning exercises seem to promote a greater abstract reasoning reserve, and so on. I have a physician friend, Dr. Roger Kendrick, who is so sure that constantly challenging your brain with new types of learning prevents dementia and keeps you sharp, that he started learning Chinese a few years ago. I saw him at a meeting recently and asked him if he felt the intense process of learning all those Chinese ideographs had actually helped him, and he said he was positive that he was mentally sharper now than he had ever been in his life.

How to Do Them

Like a physical-exercise program, the purpose of a brain-exercise program is first, to ensure regularity, and second, to use those muscles (i.e., cognitive functions) that are not commonly used in normal life as one currently lives it. If, say, you read the newspaper cover-to-cover daily, you are already giving one group of cognitive functions a nice workout—in particular, the functions of symbol-decoding and abstract reasoning. Whether or not this routine also exercises your short-term memory depends on what you do with the information you read. After reading an article—particularly one that interests you—do you do anything that tests your retention of what you have read? Probably not, or at least not until later when you are telling a friend about the article, and realize that you have to check back to see if you have the facts right. Here, then, is a good example of a simple add-on exercise you can do when reading the paper:

Brain Exercise 1

ALL THE NEWS THAT FITS

After reading the newspaper, turn back to the first page and pick out a headline of one of the articles that you have read to the end. Now fold the paper closed and see how much of the article you can recall. The names of the principal people in the article? Any figures mentioned in it—numbers, percentages, rates, and so on? Check back and see how you did.

If you challenge yourself to this little quiz on a regular basis, you will soon notice that you are reading the paper with greater care, automatically making an effort to commit more of it to memory, and hence retaining more and more of what you have read. Such a daily workout of your short-term memory will pay off in enhanced general function of short-term memory.

I particularly like these exercises that add on to some routine that is already part of your life. It is a bit like holding hand weights during your regular walk to the train station.

Another add-on exercise for short-term memory function is:

Brain Exercise 2

TV QUIZ

After watching the TV news, turn off the set and simply see how many of the individual stories that were broadcast you can list on a piece of paper—just the general topic, not the full idea. Incredibly, most adults can only recall half of the news stories they have seen immediately after the program is over. So much for the lasting impact of the Information Age! (This, like other brain tests and exercises, requires a partner who jots down the programs as they are shown; some couples I know alternate being tester and testee from evening to evening.)

As with the newspaper quiz, you will find yourself meeting the challenge by attending better and remembering more, a good workout for memorizing information that you have processed in a different way. You can up the ante by adding commercials to the items you attempt to play back after the show is over.

Another popular add-on brain exercise is:

Brain Exercise 3

PHOTOGRAPH RECALL

If you regularly leaf through a photo magazine like *National Geographic,* you can ask your partner to test your memory of the details in a particular photograph or group of photographs. What is the number of people pictured, the color of a shirt, what was written on a street sign, and so on?

Again, the memory of an image tests and exercises short-term memory of information that has been mentally processed in yet a different way from information acquired by reading or listening. Some people resist exercises like these because they are afraid of clogging up their memories with useless information. They think of the brain as a cup that can only hold so much and then starts spilling over, indiscriminately expelling valuable information along with useless information in the overflow.

Not so. Information that you consciously and unconsciously deem valuable gets downloaded into long-term memory, while all the rest is dumped at regular intervals. Overloading does not figure into this. On the contrary, the very point is that the more you use your short-term memory, the more it will develop and hold in the future.

There is another group of short-term memory exercises that I favor because the exercises are so easily integrated into a regular routine. They do not qualify as add-ons, strictly speaking, but they do involve activities that are already part of your day.

Brain Exercise 4

NUMBER-STRING RETENTION

Pick a series of one- and two-digit numbers from the newspaper. You can find loads of these in the financial section (shares sold, opening quotes, currency conversions), and in the weather section (temperatures, humidity, or rainfall in major cities). Start by studying a string of five such numbers for three minutes. Test yourself. If you remember them all, add another number to the string, study for another two minutes, and test yourself again. Keep adding numbers to the string until you are unable to remember the complete list. An hour later, test yourself again to see how many of the numbers in the string you retain.

This is a particularly good test for systematically measuring your improvement with regular mental exercise. As well, it is a reliable way for you to judge the effectiveness of any nootropics you are experimenting with. If, say, after taking 150 milligrams of Gingko biloba daily for three months you are still only able to play back the same amount of numbers in the string as when you started with the supplement, you may want to either increase your dosage of the Gingko biloba or use a different nootropic.

Brain Exercises in Popular Culture

Popular culture, famous for polluting our brains, also offers us several highly effective and easily accessible brain exercises in the form of word puzzles and video games. The former chiefly exercise perception, verbal skills, and abstract reasoning; the latter primarily exercise attention, reflexes, and eye-hand coordination. Both the puzzles and the games are entertaining (after all, that's the main reason people buy them), and tend to be arranged in order of increasing difficulty, perfect for developing a cognitive faculty by increments over a period of time.

Word Puzzle Brain Exercises

The most effective among these are Word Mazes: a page covered with columns of seemingly random letters in which words are hidden, forward, backward, vertically, horizontally, and diagonally. Popular items for bus and subway commuters, books of these mazes can be bought in most news shops. They give your eye-perception faculty a real workout. Anagram puzzles, sometimes called Jumbles, are also effective and popular word puzzles. In these, a common word is given with the letters out of sequence; timing yourself, you have to come up with that word—a great workout for perception, verbal skills, and abstract reasoning. Like other brain exercises, these puzzles can be done regularly in down time such as when traveling or in waiting rooms. Best to time yourself when doing them, both to put pressure on your brain to work faster (similar in a way to aerobic exercise), and to measure your progress.

In general, the most popular and intellectual of word puzzles, crossword puzzles, are the least effective for exercising your brain. They tend to put to greater emphasis on long-term memory-information retrieval than on perception or reasoning. And, by and large, of all of our cognitive functions, long-term memory is the least affected by aging.

The puzzle section of any large bookstore offers an ever-changing supply of all kinds of puzzle books with names like Brain Teasers or IQ, that can challenge a variety of cognitive functions including spatial-relations reasoning, logical thinking, and structuralization, in addition to memory, perception, and verbal reasoning. In general, look for those puzzle books that emphasize skills such as these as compared to Trivial Pursuit-like information games and puzzles.

Video Game Brain Exercises

I can already hear some of you protesting the idea that video games could possibly be good for the health and plasticity of your brain, but indeed, these games offer highly productive and efficient training for your attention/perception, reflex, and coordination faculties—all of them faculties that tend to diminish with age if they are not exercised regularly.

First, I should assure you that there are many video games out there that do not revolve around ugly, aggressive pursuits like airplane battles or kung-fu fights. One of my favorites is innocent to the point of being positively whimsical; it is Glider, in which the player uses a mouse or keyboard to keep a toy glider aloft by avoiding collisions and guiding it to updrafts. It requires quick perception and response; it is constructed for increasing, graduated difficulty; and it is played against time with a scoring system that measures improvement. There is an ever-expanding array of perception-and-response video games. These involve a variety of visio-spatial (including 3-D) and structural skills. Check them out in any software store or catalog.

Spending fifteen to twenty minutes a day exercising your brain with video games has been conclusively demonstrated to measurably improve perception/reaction time in adults. Your first problem, of course, is getting them away from any resident (or visiting) child.

College Prep Revisited

There is nothing quite so humbling as looking back at college entrance tests and the courses you may have taken in preparation for these tests at the age of seventeen or eighteen. Did I ever really know how to do this stuff? is the question that most often springs to mind. The answer, of course, is Yes. What's more, you are now probably as able (if not more so) to perform well on these tests as you were back then. But you have to get back in mental shape to do so. And for revitalizing the cognitive faculties of abstract and logical reasoning, short- and long-term memory, and verbal and arithmetic thinking, the home preparatory courses for these tests have no equal. In particular, I recommend those courses that you can use on a computer, complete with timed tests.

And Now For Something Really New

The brain exercises discussed above pay off in increased cognitive function, but not in immediate practical application of content. The final category of exercise will do both: setting ourselves the task of learning an area of new knowledge from the ground up. Such a challenge can be done alone or in an adult classroom and may be a new language, a new computer skill, a new fine motor skill like woodcarving, even an in-depth study of some subject that has always attracted you, like military insignia of the First World War, or Norse mythology. And few things are more likely to make you feel youthful than some interesting new knowledge.

The two keys to any brain exercise program you set for yourself are regularity and variety. Even if you can only allot fifteen minutes a day to these exercises—say, while you are on the commuter train or aboard your exercise bicycle—the fact that you give your brain a steady workout will still pay off. And just as cross-training of a variety of muscle groups brings you the best total results in physical exercise, cross-training of different cognitive functions will give you the best total results in brain exercises.

PART IV
❧
Mega-Chicken Soup

*T*he effects of a strengthened immune system are primarily experienced as double negatives: no interminable infections, no debilitating viral diseases, no deadly cancer. A person who has boosted his ability to fend off his body's foreign invaders and to, say, detect newly formed cancer cells before they do major mischief, spends longer periods free of disease than he did before, and would normally, as he grows older. But how does this double negative translate into subjective experience?

A person who had been suffering for years from chronic bronchial infections will certainly take notice when he suddenly finds himself free of them for an entire winter. He will feel this absence of disease as the presence of higher energy and better spirits. And that is precisely the kind of outcome one can expect when he goes on a regime of strong antioxidants, hormone supplements, physical exercise, and stress-reduction techniques.

The Been-Sick-So-Long-It-Feels-Like-Normal-to-Me Blues

Chronic infections can become so much a part of an individual's life that she accepts it as normal, especially if that person lives a

IMMUNE SYSTEM ECONOMICS

Is it starting to occur to you that the costs of thoroughly engaging in the Triple-Your-Youthspan Program could start to add up?

True, many of these supplements are far from cheap, especially when taken regularly in potent dosages, but consider the alternatives *in purely economic terms.* I am referring to lost income due to sick days, and to the decreased efficiency (and therefore, income) due to the decline in energy experienced by people with chronic low-grade infections. And I am referring to the cost of office visits to the doctor, cold and other over-the-counter preparations, and prescription drugs that you would inevitably incur if you were to fall victim to common infections.

My point is simple: the dollars-and-cents bottom line is that taking the supplements available to you today that build a strong immune system is a major bargain.

highly pressured lifestyle. Such a person can come to think of her relentless cough, sinus infections, and psoriasis as simply a part of aging that she has to endure but cannot pay too much attention to because she simply doesn't have the time. When these complaints become overwhelming, she heads for her doctor, who prescribes various antibiotics that probably become decreasingly effective with each passing year. Obviously, this course of action does nothing to prevent such infections from occurring in the first place. And it certainly does nothing to extend her Youthspan.

People with high-stress jobs often have low immune functioning as a result of all the stress hormones they are constantly producing. So one logical step in a program to build up their immune system is to try to reduce those stress hormones at their source by lowering overall stress. That is why meditation, visualization, and physical exercise are part of my program. In addition, anything else that reduces stress for you—say, a massage or an hour in a flotation tank—should be seriously considered as part of your personal program. Remember, these practices not only make you feel better, they build your resistance to a broad spectrum of diseases.

A PREVENTATIVE-MEDICINE DOCTOR'S APPROACH

If a person suffering from chronic infections consults a doctor of preventative medicine, he may start by measuring various of his patient's immune parameters, such as his total levels of different types of T-cells, his immunoglobulin response to certain vaccines, and his plasma cortisol and zinc levels. And if, say, cortisol is high (undoubtedly due to stress), and zinc is low, he can see immediately that his patient's immune system is operating at decreased capacity and needs all the help it can get.

This doctor may or may not prescribe an antibiotic to control a current infection or infections, depending on how dangerous they are. But his basic approach will be to boost his patient's immune system so that future infections will not take hold. To this end he will prescribe stress-reduction techniques, antioxidants, and various other supplements, possibly including some hormones if they appear to be in decline, as well as the immune-stimulating herb echinacea, which can be found in any health food store. In future visits, this doctor will again measure the patient's immune parameters to gauge how much they have improved and, possibly, to adjust dosages of the supplements to stimulate further improvement.

CHAPTER EIGHT

Basic Mega-Chicken Soup Tools I: Supplements

Antioxidants—The Big Picture

*I*t is abundantly clear to all of us in the youth extension business that one of our prime tasks is to do battle with free radicals of all types. Our basic weapons in this war are reducing exposure to substances that generate free radicals in our bodies (mainly cigarette smoke, excess alcohol, and environmental toxins), and using antioxidants, from both food sources and supplements. Each of these can significantly retard the rate of cellular death, thus promoting a much longer, disease-free Youthspan.

I promised at the outset to separate health-food fads from well-tested strategies for preserving youth. Well, antioxidants are definitely the real thing. Even mainstream medicine has finally acknowledged this fact—the evidence in the scientific literature has become just too overwhelming not to.

Most folks (myself included) would prefer to obtain their antioxidant nutrients solely through their diets. But the fact is that a sufficiently antioxidant-rich diet would require such vigilant monitoring of our daily food intake that few people would—or could—actually maintain it. We would have to weigh each portion of food and calculate its content for a variety of nutrients, taking into account where the food was grown or raised and, in some cases, in what season. For example, the selenium content of vegetables varies with the density of selenium in the soil where the vegetables are grown, and this can deviate from one area to another by a considerable degree. Testing plasma antioxidant levels of people who consume relatively healthy diets (or who think they do) shows that many still have relatively low levels of carotenoids, tocopherols, and other critical natural antioxidants; in short, these health-conscious people are not getting adequate amounts of antioxidants to lengthen their Youthspans. For this reason, supplements are a basic part of my program.

Antioxidants basically come in three forms: vitamins that work directly as antioxidants; minerals that work as cofactors within anti-oxidant enzyme systems present in our cells; and nonvitamin and nonmineral compounds that work as antioxidants. These include substances like flavonoids found in fruits and vegetables, and certain compounds our bodies make, such as uric acid and melatonin.

A word about dosages: The scientific literature is full of research suggesting that the government's "daily allowances" (DAs) for many vitamins and minerals are too low for optimal health. That's because these government-issued DAs are based predominantly on research which suggest that these are the amounts you need daily to avoid a "deficiency" disease of that vitamin. For example, eating at least sixty milligrams of vitamin C daily (the current DA) will keep you from getting scurvy. But is sixty milligrams enough to actually give an adult optimal health, in addition to preventing the development of scurvy? Many studies have suggested it is not.

The same may be true for vitamin E. There is now a vast amount of research which indicates that supplemental vitamin E is a safe and effective way to prevent coronary artery disease, when given in doses far above its current DA. In addition, a recent study also showed that people sixty-five and over generated a significantly greater antibody response to both hepatitis B and tetanus vaccines if they had been taking a supplement of vitamin E that was around six times its DA for four months.

One final introductory note: aerobic exercise, which is an important element in the Triple-Your Youthspan Program, can result in the generation of free radicals, particularly in our muscle cells. But research shows that using oral antioxidants can minimize this free-radical damage in our muscle cells as a result of regular exercise.

For example, people taking vitamin E supplements have been shown to generate less free-radical tissue damage during aerobic exercise than those who are not.

Beta Carotene and the Carotenoids

WHAT THEY ARE AND HOW THEY WORK

Beta carotene and other carotenoids are lipid-soluble compounds that a plant makes to protect itself from the oxygen free radicals generated by photosynthesis. Many of the carotenoids can be converted to limited amounts of vitamin A in the human body after they have been absorbed in the intestine, but they also contribute to an extended Youthspan in ways that are unrelated to their conversion to vitamin A.

In addition to beta carotene, the carotenoids found most prevalently in our blood serum are lycopene, beta cryptoxanthin, lutein, zeaxanthin, and alpha carotene. Like vitamins and minerals, they get there entirely via our diets and supplements; the human body cannot manufacture them.

It was discovered around thirty years ago that beta carotene could squelch the dangerous superoxide anion free radicals, and it is now known that all of the carotenoids found in our plasma neutralize different types of age- and disease-promoting free radicals. Beta carotene has been the most studied carotenoid, and it is the one that you undoubtedly have heard the most about; but actually it is not the most efficient antioxidant among the carotenoids—lycopene is.

Because the carotenoids are fat-soluble compounds, they are found in the highest concentrations within the outer cell membrane itself, as well as the cell membranes that surround the various organelles within our cells, such as the mitochondria. This is where they work to prevent lipid peroxidation by oxygen free radicals.

Like many supplements with strong credentials as preventative medicine, beta carotene has come in for a great deal of criticism from the champions of disease-cure medicine. Much of the criticism, however, is backed up by clinical studies that were, in effect, designed to fail. For example, several studies were designed to see if beta carotene supplementation could be directly shown to prevent cancer from developing in people who were already at *high risk for it.*

In one of the best known of these studies, the Alpha Tocopherol—Beta Carotene (ATBC) study, cancer researchers recruited over 29,000 Finnish men with the average age of fifty-seven who had been smoking an average of a pack of cigarettes a day for almost thirty-six years. These men were then split into four groups; one group began taking twenty milligrams of beta carotene each day, another group began taking fifty milligrams of alpha tocopherol (vitamin E) a day, a third group took both, and the final group got a placebo. In the next five to eight years, 474 men in the group taking beta carotene developed lung cancer compared to 402 men who were not taking beta carotene. This caused the researchers to suggest that not only does beta carotene appear to be useless in preventing lung cancer in smokers, but that it may actually increase the risk of lung cancer in smokers as well!

Another of these studies, the Beta Carotene and Retinol Efficacy Trial (CARET), supplemented thousands of people for around four years with both beta carotene and retinol (an active form of vitamin A). Again, only *smokers, former smokers, and workers exposed to asbestos* were studied. In fact, the asbestos workers had to have a chest X-ray to prove that they already had asbestos-related lung disease to be eligible for the study.

To demonstrate that beta carotene (or anything else for that matter) will not protect a person from getting lung cancer if he takes it after years of smoking, or asbestos exposure, is not a newsflash to anyone. The precancerous changes that were destined to become cancer were already too well advanced in these individuals. Even the researchers in the ATBC trial wrote in their discussion that "it is plausible that the intervention period was too short to inhibit the development of cancers resulting from a lifetime of exposure to cigarette smoke and other carcinogens."

The real message is clear: Don't Smoke! Unfortunately, another message is obscured by these studies: *that people who are* nonsmokers *do benefit from the use of beta carotene in terms of preventing cancer.*

There are dozens of studies showing that when animals are exposed to a known cancer-causing agent, giving them beta carotene reduces or prevents the appearance of cancer. A computer search of the medical literature over the past twenty years, using "beta carotene" and "cancer" as keywords, will provide you with a long list of these studies.

A 1992 review paper published in the journal *Cancer Research* by Dr. Regina Zeigler of the National Cancer Institute summarized several previously published studies in humans in which the levels of various carotenoids in the plasma, and the incidence of cancer were followed over several years. In many of these studies, a reduction in lung, stomach, and other cancers was found in those people who had high blood levels of either beta carotene or total carotenoids. In addition, the author examined several epidemiological studies which showed a decreased incidence of cancer of several types in people with high intakes of fruits and vegetables, which are high in the carotenoids.

However, what I find particularly interesting is that just one year before the publication of the ATBC trial (which, along with the results of the CARET trial, were paraded onto the nightly news broadcasts with all sorts of "See, we-told-you-it-wouldn't-work" comments by the conventional medicine community), the September 15, 1993, issue of the *Journal of the National Cancer Institute* published a paper showing the results of the General Population Trial. This clinical trial was conducted in Linxian, China, which has an increased rate of certain types of cancers. In this study, thousands of Chinese people were given a combination of beta carotene, vitamin E, and selenium for over five years. This caused a significant reduction in the incidence of the cancer death rate in those people taking these compounds. In addition, over 3,000 other people in Linxian who had esophageal dysplasia (a precancerous condition of the esophagus) were given either a placebo or a multivitamin supplement plus beta carotene. There was a modest reduction (8 percent decline) in esophageal cancer in people taking the multivitamin and beta carotene compared to those getting the placebo.

DOSAGE

The carotenes rank high as potent and inexpensive antioxidants, and therefore are prime elements of my program. Let me first suggest that you maximize your intake of the carotenoids through foods, because foods are most likely to give you the best mix of all the carotenoids. For example, it was recently shown that people who were put on a diet of large amounts of sweet potatoes, cooked kale, and tomato juice were able to more than double their plasma levels of beta carotene, and to increase their plasma lutein and lycopene levels by 67 percent and 26 percent, respectively. This resulted in a 33 percent increase in the responsiveness of their T-cells (special immune system cells), which play a vital role in the response to foreign invaders and cancer cells. Other foods known to be among the highest in carotenoids (particularly beta carotene, lutein, and lycopene) are carrots, cantaloupe, apricots, celery, mustard greens, Brussels sprouts, green peas, scallions, peaches, Swiss chard, winter squash, red pepper, pink grapefruit, guava, watermelon, and spinach.

Even if you eat a diet high in carotenoids, you should take a supplement that contains *fifteen to twenty milligrams of beta carotene and from fifty to 100 milligrams of mixed carotenoids every other day.* Double this supplementation if you do not eat a lot of foods high in carotenoids, that is *thirty to forty milligrams of beta carotene and from 100 to 200 milligrams of mixed carotenoids every other day.* (If you smoke, drink moderately, or are overweight, you should take these supplements every day instead of every other day.) Try to take a vitamin-E supplement along with your carotenoid supplement. These supplements are available at most health food stores.

There is no danger of toxicity; doses of up to 180 milligrams of beta carotene a day for many years are well tolerated. But too much beta carotene can produce a yellowish tint in your skin, indicating large amounts of it are being deposited there; if this occurs, do not be concerned, just cut back on your intake.

Vitamin E and the Tocopherols

WHAT THEY ARE AND HOW THEY WORK

Vitamin E is the collective term for a large group of biologically active compounds made by plants that are known as tocopherols and tocotrienols. Our own cells do not manufacture these compounds, but it is clear from years of research that vitamin E plays a major role in our bodies as an antioxidant (it does the same thing in plants, protecting them from the oxygen free radicals produced during photosynthesis). Since vitamin E is fat soluble, it dissolves into all cell membranes, and that is where it does its work as an antioxidant. This is extremely significant, given the fact that oxygen free radicals cause lipid peroxidation in the cell membranes, which you now know about. Specifically, it is the polyunsaturated fatty acids in our cell membranes that take a big hit from oxygen free radicals.

One of the most highly researched effects of vitamin E is its role in preventing oxidation of low density lipoprotein (LDL) cholesterol in our blood. When LDL cholesterol is oxidized, it tends to stick to the lining of our arteries more readily than it does normally, contributing highly to the arterial blockage process known as atherosclerosis. When the arteries being blocked go to the head, a form of dementia occurs. When the arteries being blocked go to the penis, impotence results. And when the arteries being blocked are the coronary arteries, blood flow to the heart muscle is reduced and irreversible ischemic heart disease occurs.

One of my filing cabinets is now overflowing with research papers demonstrating that people taking supplements of vitamin E have a dramatically decreased risk of heart attacks caused by ischemic heart disease. For example, a 1996 study of nearly 35,000 postmenopausal women found that those women with the highest intakes of vitamin E had the lowest risk of death from coronary heart disease. Even more recently, Dr. Morris Brown of Cambridge University in England reported that in a study of 2,000 patients with existing heart disease, taking vitamin E supplements reduced the subsequent risk of both fatal and nonfatal heart attacks by a dramatic 47 and 77 percent respectively. Studies such as these have led the president of the American Heart Association, Dr. Jan Breslow, to declare recently that vitamin E, either in supplements or in food, appears to prevent coronary heart disease.

What is more, there is now strong evidence that vitamin E may protect your brain over time as well. Studies in animals show that vitamin E blocks the ability of the beta amyloid protein (the protein that forms the plaques in the brains of Alzheimer's victims) to kill neurons. It also has been shown to decrease lipofuscin accumulating in the brains of aging animals, and to prevent protein oxidation in the brain, due to free radicals. In addition, vitamin E is now known to enhance immune function in humans.

DOSAGE

Most of the studies showing benefits of vitamin E use d-alpha to-copherol, the most potent natural form of vitamin E, which is available everywhere (d,l-alpha tocopherol also works, but it has more of the inactive form of vitamin E than the d-alpha tocopherol). Doses ranging from *400 to 800 international units (IUs) per day* have been shown to be effective. This dose of vitamin E will also enter your brain cells, and will work in their cell membranes to fight against the lipid and protein oxidation that can result in cognitive problems many years down the road. (Some manufacturers label their vitamin E in milligrams, instead of IUs; one milligram of d-alpha tocopherol is equivalent to about 1.50 IUs, so if you want to take the equivalent of 400 IUs of d-alpha tocopherol, you would take around 267 milligrams.)

It is difficult to get this amount of vitamin E from foods without also taking in a lot of fat because vitamin E is mostly present in fatty foods like nuts. It is also present in some nonfatty green, leafy vegetables, like spinach; however, it has been estimated that you would need to eat nineteen cups of spinach to ingest just 100 IUs of vitamin E, a tall order even for the likes of Popeye. Therefore, the supplements appear to be a much more practical source.

If you do not eat large quantities of fruits and vegetables that are high in vitamin C, you should take a vitamin-C supplement with your vitamin E, as they work synergistically in reducing free radical damage. However, if you have a vitamin K deficiency, or you are currently using Warfarin or other blood-thinning drugs, you should consult your physician prior to taking vitamin E supplements.

Vitamin C

WHAT IT IS AND HOW IT WORKS

Unlike most mammals, humans do not manufacture vitamin C (L-ascorbic acid)—we lack the enzyme gulonolactone oxidase, that is needed to make it. A failure to acquire vitamin C in our diet results in the fairly rapid onset of specific disease symptoms, such as abnormal sensitivity to heat and cold, bleeding gums, easy bruising, glaucoma, cataracts, depression, and a host of others. In the eighteenth century, English sailors under the command of Captain James

Cook, who were at sea for months at a time without fresh fruits or vegetables (prime sources of vitamin C), discovered that sucking on limes prevented them from getting scurvy (which is how they acquired the nickname "limeys"). Today, vitamin C is the most commonly used supplement in the United States.

Vitamin C is critical in the synthesis of collagen, a substance that helps to cement our cells together. But it is also one of the most powerful oxygen free radical scavengers available to our bodies. Unlike vitamin E, which is fat soluble, C is water soluble and so does its work in the cell's plasma and watery interior (cytosol). But vitamin C is also extremely effective at protecting the cell membrane by scooping up free radicals in the cytosol and so preventing them from moving into the cell membrane and initiating lipid peroxidation. Evidence also suggests that vitamin C plays an important role in preventing cancer. Finally, the vitamin has been found to regenerate the protective form of vitamin E and other antioxidants that have made their way to the cell membrane; for this reason it is a natural complement to vitamin E.

DOSAGE

Ever since Linus Pauling's suggestion that megadoses of vitamin C (up to sixteen grams daily) could prevent the common cold, the debate has raged about the optimum dosage of this common vitamin. At the other end of the spectrum are scientists who maintain that a vitamin-C concentration range in the plasma of forty to sixty micromolar is all that is needed for good health. This level can be achieved in most people by ingesting 100 to 150 milligrams of vitamin C daily. My educated guess is that it lies somewhere in between, though quite a bit higher than the low end. After looking at the most recent studies, including one done by the National Institutes of Health, I believe all healthy adults should be consuming between *500 and 1,000 milligrams a day* of vitamin C. I have read the arguments about vitamin C stimulating the formation of kidney stones, but this seems extremely unlikely at this dose.

If you have chronic infections (which can result in the loss of vitamin C), you should take up to *2,000 milligrams* (two grams) *a day*. (First check with your doctor to make sure you are not taking any drugs which could be rendered inactive by vitamin C supplements.) If you smoke, drink alcohol even moderately, or use oral contraceptives, you should take 1.5 to 2.0 grams of vitamin C daily. I do not recommend taking megadoses (several grams), because such high doses can interact with free iron in your body and actually *produce* free radicals instead of squelching them. In addition, you should not take vitamin C within two hours before or after meals high in heme iron (which is the type of iron found in a meat meal) if you already have high iron stores; that is because vitamin C increases the absorption of iron from your intestine, even if your body does not need it, and excessive body-iron stores have now been correlated with an increased risk of several diseases, including heart disease.

Glutathione

WHAT IT IS AND HOW IT WORKS

As an antioxidant, glutathione (GSH) is one of the most important substances in my program. A small tripeptide (composed of three amino acids) found in all our cells, GSH performs as an antioxidant by detoxifying hydrogen peroxide into water molecules before it can be transformed into a dangerous hydroxyl free radical. This decreases the long-term risk of cancer, heart disease, and other degenerative diseases. This antioxidant action of GSH is catalyzed (sped up) by the selenium-containing enzyme, glutathione peroxidase (GPX).

GSH is important in all cells, particularly so in our livers. We are exposed to different toxins every day—for example, the average American is exposed to fourteen pounds of food additives each year, many of which are toxic, and when these toxins enter our bodies, our livers activate the cytochrome P-450 enzymes. These enzymes then convert the toxic compounds to less toxic substances that can be excreted out of the body (this process is called the "phase-I" liver reaction).

Phase-I liver reactions also create large amounts of free radicals; therefore, in what is known as the phase-II reactions in the liver, GSH and other antioxidants neutralize them. If you have a lot of oxidative stress (due to excess exposure to environmental toxins, or if you are a smoker or drink alcohol excessively), your phase-I liver enzymes are working overtime. And if your phase-I enzymes are working hard, your phase-II reactions had better be up to the task (which means having lots of GSH around), or the result may eventually be liver damage due to excess generation of free radicals.

GSH is probably even working on toxic substances in your diet before they reach your liver. That is because in mammals it seems to be present in the cells that line the intestine, which are the first line of defense against toxic compounds being absorbed into the body. More importantly, these cells seem to be able to take up GSH and use it to protect against toxins entering the blood. This was clearly shown in a study in which these special intestinal epithelial cells were isolated from rats and GSH was added to the medium; when GSH was added twenty minutes before a highly toxic, oxidizing compound was introduced, the intestinal cells were protected against the damaging effects of the toxin. If these cells do become damaged, toxic substances in your diet can be absorbed and enter your bloodstream. Some physicians call this the "leaky-gut syndrome," which plays a role in the onset of many chronic illnesses, such as Crohn's disease and rheumatoid arthritis.

DOSAGE

There are three ways to increase the amount of GSH your body has available; you can increase your intake of foods high in GSH, you can take GSH supplements (available as L-GSH in stores, the biologically active isomer of GSH; however, I will continue to refer to it here as simply GSH), or you can take supplements of the amino acid L-cysteine, which results in increased synthesis of GSH in our cells. Although it is a small peptide, oral GSH supplements have been clearly shown to be absorbed intact in humans.

Vegetables high in GSH are: avocados, carrots, tomatoes, lettuce, green peppers, asparagus, raw spinach, okra, broccoli, potatoes, squash, and cauliflower. Citrus fruits, as well as strawberries, watermelon, and fresh peaches are also relatively high in glutathione. However, I cannot recommend relying on food sources of GSH alone, because the amount of GSH found in foods varies significantly, depending on where it was grown, and how it was prepared (GSH can be destroyed by cooking).

Taking L-cysteine supplements, which are quite inexpensive, is an excellent way to boost your cellular GSH levels. The best supplement form of it seems to be N-acetyl-L-cysteine (NAC) capsules, which are available in most health food stores, and the supplement sources noted in the Resources section. I have read several human clinical studies showing that NAC increases the activity and effectiveness of GPX, and NAC has been used to treat chronic lung diseases for around thirty years (it helps break up mucus). A recent study shows that NAC significantly blocks the oxidation of plasma proteins by cigarette smoke in cigarette smokers; imagine what it might do for you if you don't smoke.

The recommended *daily dose of GSH is 100 to 200 milligrams.* However, if you eat lots of foods high in GSH, I would only take 100 to 200 milligrams every other day or use NAC instead, as I and many others do. The effective daily dose of NAC seems to be around 500 to 600 milligrams.

Two cofactors you should take to maximize the effectiveness of your body's GSH are alpha lipoic acid (ALA), and selenium. ALA is important in recycling GSH from its oxidized to its reduced form, so it can continue to work for you (see below); and selenium, because the enzyme GPX is what allows GSH to function adequately. GPX, in turn, requires selenium to work efficiently.

Therefore, along with my NAC, I personally take *100 milligrams of ALA and 200 micrograms of selenium, every other day.* You can buy all of these products separately, but if you want to take an all-in-one combination, Douglas Laboratories (listed in the Resources section) manufactures a product known as GSH 250 Master Glutathione Formula, which contains 250 milligrams of GSH and NAC, along with 200 milligrams of ALA and 25 micrograms of selenium. If you eat large quantities of GSH-containing foods, this lab also makes Glutaplex, which is the same as GSH 250 Master Glutathione Formula except that it contains only 50 milligrams each of NAC, GSH, and ALA.

It may also be a good idea to take supplements of curcumin along with GSH. Curcumin is a natural phenolic substance derived from turmeric, the spice that gives curry its yellow color. Curcumin has long been recognized as a potent antioxidant in its own right. However, part of its antioxidant reputation may be derived from the fact that it augments the expression and function of GSH.

Alpha Lipoic Acid

WHAT IT IS AND HOW IT WORKS

Alpha lipoic acid (ALA), also called thioctic acid, is a cofactor for the pyruvate dehydrogenase complex in the mitochondrial matrix. Put more simply, this means that it is critical in allowing the mitochondria to manufacture needed cell energy in the form of ATP. ALA has been shown in several studies to enhance certain forms of memory, so it makes a nice addition to any nootropic program. But I list it here because ALA is yet another safe compound with very potent antioxidant properties. It works in both the lipid-cell membranes as well as the cytosol of cells to effectively scavenge several types of oxygen free radicals. In addition, ALA has been shown to protect LDL cholesterol against oxidation, reducing the threat of atherosclerosis.

ALA also appears to have a number of beneficial effects both in prevention of and therapy for diabetes. If your glucose levels remain high for excessive periods of time (common in Type-II diabetes and in Type-I diabetics who fail to take their insulin shots when they should), the glucose reacts with proteins in what is called a "glycation" reaction that can result in serious damage to our cells and is believed to be responsible for many of the health problems associated with both Type-I and -II diabetes. This is one of the reasons your physician is likely to put you on synthetic drugs to try and lower your glucose levels when you have Type-II diabetes. However, ALA has been shown to prevent glycation reactions in diabetics who do not use these synthetic drugs.

DOSAGE

Normal healthy individuals can benefit from ALA by taking *100 to 200 milligrams either every day or every other day*. If you take different vitamins and nutrients on different days, take your ALA on the same days as your GSH and vitamins E and C, because it helps recycle them back into their effective antioxidant form.

If you are a Type-I or Type-II diabetic, you should take a total of 400 or 500 milligrams of ALA daily, divided up with your meals (for example, if you have two major meals a day, take 200 to 250 milligrams with each meal). After a month of taking ALA daily, monitor your blood-glucose levels immediately after meals to see if you can begin taking less insulin if you are a Type-I diabetic, or less of any glucose-lowering drugs you may be using if you are a Type-II diabetic.

Coenzyme Q10

WHAT IT IS AND HOW IT WORKS

Ubiquinones are compounds that allow ATP synthesis to occur, participating in the transfer of electrons in the mitochondria. ATP is the cell's energy currency; as it is not stored in the cell, the cell has to manufacture it continuously in the mitochondria. If the cell runs low on ATP, it cannot do the energy-requiring things it needs to do to stay healthy, and if it runs very low on ATP, it dies.

A ubiquinone that can be readily synthesized in the laboratory goes by the name of coenzyme Q10, and it is one of the most potent and underrated Youthspan extenders currently available in your pharmacy or health food store. One of the beneficial effects of coenzyme Q10 is seen in patients with mitochondrial disease (diseases in which the primary problem is that the mitochondria are damaged, and therefore not producing adequate amounts of cellular energy). Many victims of mitochondrial disease have reportedly shown significant improvement when given coenzyme Q10 supplements. But more importantly in terms of my program, ongoing studies indicate that regular supplements of coenzyme Q10 in healthy individuals reduce the likelihood of contracting these mitochondrial diseases in the first place.

Coenzyme Q10 has also been shown to have a dramatic effect on cardiovascular function in humans, particularly in its ability to protect the heart during periods when it is deprived of oxygen, and a pronounced benefit in preventing atherosclerosis (clogging of the arteries). As we have seen, vitamin E squelches the oxygen free radicals that oxidize plasma LDL molecules. But in another one of the body's can't-win-for-losing mechanisms, the vitamin E sometimes takes on an extra electron during this reaction, and becomes a free radical itself. Research shows, however, that when coenzyme Q10 is present in the blood in adequate amounts, it quickly transforms vitamin E back into its stable, antioxidant form, so that it can continue to do its job, and not cause any problems of its own. Thus, coenzyme Q10 supplements should be taken along with vitamin-E supplements if the vitamin E is to work most efficiently.

As elevated blood pressure is one of the greatest risk factors for the onset of heart disease and stroke in middle age, another way coenzyme Q10 guards against a reduced Youthspan is through its regulation of blood pressure. A recent clinical study of more than one hundred patients with hypertension showed that when these patients were given daily doses of coenzyme Q10 in addition to their regular blood pressure medications, a very high percentage were able to safely reduce their dosage of the medication within six months.

Amazingly, 51 percent of them were able to completely stop taking the hypertensive drugs they had been using within an average of 4.4 months after starting to take coenzyme Q10. This not only meant that these patients were no longer at risk for the side effects of their hypertensive drugs—a daunting list that includes impotence and chronic depression—but it also meant significant economic savings for them.

DOSAGE

Based on a variety of studies, a safe and effective oral dose of coenzyme Q10 for healthy people over the age of thirty is between *50 and 100 milligrams daily*. A large study of normal, disease-free subjects showed a significant increase in blood levels of coenzyme Q10 when they took an oral dose of ninety milligrams daily.

People with certain diseases appear to benefit from higher doses. For example, one study of women with breast cancer who received the relatively high dose of 390 milligrams per day along with conventional therapy experienced a significantly greater reduction of tumors spreading to the lung cavities and liver than those who only received the conventional therapy. In another study, over half of patients with essential hypertension (high blood pressure of unknown cause) receiving an average dose of 225 milligrams of coenzyme Q10 daily, along with prescription blood-pressure medications, were able to stop taking their prescription antihypertensives within just ten weeks.

If you can find coenzyme Q10 in soft gelatin tablets with only soybean oil mixed in, that may be your best buy. A recent study of four different preparations of the substance in healthy volunteers indicated that coenzyme Q10 packed this way was the most bioavailable (efficiently absorbed) source of it.

Although supplementation with coenzyme Q10 is in itself a good and safe idea, we should also try to maximize our body's own production of it. Therefore, coenzyme Q10 should be taken along with vitamin B6 (pyridoxal), which is essential for our bodies to synthesize maximal amounts of its own coenzyme Q10.

Pycnogenol

WHAT IT IS AND HOW IT WORKS

Although it is relatively unknown outside of the European scientific community, Pycnogenol is one of the most potent antioxidants you can currently purchase. Another "natural miracle," it is an extract of the maritime pine tree, which grows on the coast of France and contains a composite of forty natural compounds, including the pro-anthocyanidins (PACS). These have been shown to be more effective than either vitamin C or vitamin E as antioxidants, when given in the same concentrations.

Grape-seed extract has also been found to contain significant quantities of the same potent antioxidants found in Pycnogenol, namely the PACS. The makers of Pycnogenol claim that their PACS are more potent antioxidants than the PACS in grape-seed extract, but from the literature I have seen it appears there is very little difference in the antioxidant activity of the two. There is, however, a significant difference in their relative cost, Pycnogenol being more expensive than the grape-seed extract.

In any case, both supplements are relatively new to physicians in the United States. Anecdotal reports from those who have prescribed Pycnogenol describe cases of reduced symptoms of several chronic diseases, including autoimmune disorder, Alzheimer's, and attention deficit disorder. In addition, some research studies have demonstrated that Pycnogenol has the ability to inhibit collagenase and elastase, the enzymes which break down the proteins that are important in keeping our skin firm and young-looking (collagen and elastin, respectively).

DOSAGE

Proper dosaging of Pycnogenol involves some fairly elaborate arithmetic. First, you want to work your way up to saturation dosage over the course of ten days, and then you want to cut back to a daily maintenance dosage.

The recommended dose you want to achieve on Day Ten is about 1.4 milligrams for each pound of your body weight. In other words, if you weigh 200 pounds, you should take a gradually increasing dose over ten days until you are taking 280 milligrams (1.4 times 200) on Day Ten. The simplest way to parcel out your doses from Day One to Day Ten is to divide your Day Ten target saturation dose by ten; that becomes your dose for Day One, twice that amount is your dose for Day Two, and so on. After you have reached your saturation dose at Day Ten, you should cut your dosage in half, to around *0.7 milligrams of Pycnogenol for each pound of body weight.*

As grape-seed extract contains similar levels of the active ingredient in Pycnogenol that makes it a potent antioxidant, it is a considerably less expensive alternative. The dosage regime is similar, though.

Neither Pycnogenol nor grape-seen extract have any known toxicity in humans.

Other Important Vitamins and Minerals (Non-Antioxidants)

Selenium

WHAT IT IS AND HOW IT WORKS

Selenium acts as an antioxidant, but unlike the antioxidants listed above, it does so "indirectly." Several minerals work as cofactors in antioxidant enzymes—most prominently copper and manganese in addition to selenium—but of these, only selenium is usually missing from a normal diet. It is a cofactor within a particular antioxidant enzyme system, the glutathione peroxidase enzyme (GPX) system, which is one of the most important endogenous enzymes our cells have to control oxygen free radicals. GPX needs selenium to do its job—selenium supplements increase its antioxidant activity. And since the job of GPX is to essentially enhance the ability of the substance glutathione (GSH) to neutralize peroxides before they can be converted into free radicals, you should include GSH, or a GSH precursor along with your selenium.

For some time it has been known that giving selenium supplements to animals dramatically reduces the incidence of cancer, but now an impressive number of human clinical trials in more than twenty countries also show a significant decrease in the incidence of cancer in humans taking selenium supplements. In fact, a large, recent clinical trial in the U.S. using selenium supplements in around 1,300 people for an average of 4.5 years concluded that taking selenium supplements clearly reduced the risk of total cancer incidence and mortality in these individuals.

DOSAGE

How much selenium we have in our bodies at any given time is a function of how much selenium is in our diet (we cannot manufacture a mineral), but, of course, the selenium content of foods can vary greatly depending on the selenium content of the soil it was grown in.

The average blood level of selenium in persons in the U.S. is in the range of 1.30 to 1.80 micromoles of selenium per liter of plasma, although measurement of the activity of GPX in the blood is thought to be a better indicator of selenium status than blood-selenium levels. The average daily intake of selenium in the U.S. that produces this blood level of selenium is between 60 and 160 micrograms per day. The levels of selenium intake that have been found to be safe, and optimize the activity of GPX in humans, range from 125 to 600 micrograms per day.

For normal, healthy people, I recommend *200 micrograms every other day* (that's what I take). However, do not exceed 600 micrograms per day, as you will approach toxic blood levels.

If you are taking selenium supplements and start to experience muscle twitching, lethargy, hair loss, abdominal cramps, white streaking in your nails, or your nails falling out, you may have selenium poisoning. Stop taking the supplements, and have your plasma-selenium levels checked by your doctor. Selenium is a very important mineral for Youthspan enhancement, but you do not want to have too much of it.

You can purchase either organic or inorganic selenium, but organic selenium may be a better choice because animal studies show it inhibits cancer more effectively.

Folate/Folic Acid

WHAT IT IS AND HOW IT WORKS

Folate is a vitamin, also known as folic acid, that has many functions. One of these which has been known for some time is that it is extremely important in preventing neural-tube defects in the fetuses of pregnant women. Now, it also appears to play a significant role in preventing certain forms of heart disease, as well as colorectal cancer, the second most deadly cancer in the United States.

Indeed, when researchers look at human food intakes, they have consistently found more precancerous growths (polyps) in the colon and rectum of people with a low folate diet than in people with a diet high in folate.

I have also read a number of compelling studies that indicate that taking folate supplements provides protection against cancer of the cervix, lungs, stomach, and esophagus as well. These studies suggest that there are several ways in which insufficient folate in our bodies can lead to cancer. For example, low blood-folate levels may result in disrupted integrity of our DNA, can cause a secondary choline deficiency (which can promote some types of cancer), and may impair the natural killer cells in our immune system. Furthermore, inadequate blood levels of folate may even allow tumor-promoting viruses more easy access to our DNA.

The fact that folate supplements seem to protect us against cancer suggests that many people do not consume adequate amounts of it in their food. An excellent review paper on folate in our diets was published in 1996 by Dr. Joel Mason, at the Jean Mayer USDA Human Nutrition Research Center on Aging, at Tufts University; it's worth looking up.

Folate also seems to be important in protecting against cardiovascular disease and stroke by helping to keep that risky amino acid, homocysteine, in check (high plasma-homocysteine levels have been consistently correlated with heart disease and stroke for almost thirty years). A variety of studies show that high levels of folate in the blood are usually correlated with low levels of homocysteine, resulting in a significantly lower risk for both heart disease and stroke. Studies have also shown that the elderly, in particular, can significantly reduce their plasma-homocysteine levels by adding more folate to their diet either through foodstuffs or supplements.

The Centers for Disease Control and Prevention thinks getting more folate in our diet is so important that it has now recommended that the nation's food supply be fortified with it beginning in 1998.

DOSAGE

One of the ways to increase your plasma folate is to increase your intake of green leafy vegetables and citrus fruits. Most people, however, are unwilling to make this change in their diets, so I recommend taking folate as a supplement. Clinical trials have demonstrated that when folic-acid supplements are taken in the range of one to ten milligrams per day they provide effective prevention against several types of cancer. Smokers, who are at a higher risk for cancer to begin with, have consistently lower blood levels of folate than non-smokers, and therefore need folate supplements more than nonsmokers.

There is little evidence that folic-acid supplements are toxic, especially when given at less than five milligrams per day. Therefore, I recommend nonsmokers take *one or two milligrams of folic acid a day,* and smokers take *three to four milligrams a day.* I would also suggest taking a *vitamin B6 supplement along with your folate,* as this vitamin also plays a role in keeping your plasma-homocysteine levels low.

Caution: If you have a known vitamin B12 deficiency, or are receiving drugs for seizures or for an existing cancer, you should talk to your physician before taking folic-acid supplements. If you are a strict vegetarian, you should be tested to be sure you do not have a vitamin B12 deficiency before taking folic-acid supplements.

Zinc

WHAT IT IS AND HOW IT WORKS

Zinc is a cofactor for almost three hundred cellular enzymes, and is required for normal DNA synthesis as well as protein synthesis. It is also critical for maintaining a healthy immune system. For example, it has been shown that a zinc deficiency readily affects the proliferation and maturation of lymphocytes, very important cells of the immune system. In addition, cytokines (chemicals that cells release to regulate the immune system—interleukens, interferons, and others) require the presence of zinc to work properly. In fact, the effect of zinc on the immune system is so profound that recent studies have even shown that people taking zinc while actually having a common cold can reduce the duration of the cold. For example, a 1996 study found that people who began taking zinc lozenges containing around thirteen milligrams of zinc within twenty-four hours after developing a cold (average intake was about six lozenges per day) had fewer days with coughing, headache, hoarseness, sore throat, and nasal drainage, and a shorter overall duration of the cold when compared to people developing colds and taking placebo lozenges.

Zinc deficiency is widespread, especially in populations that subsist almost entirely on unfortified cereal grains, but inadequate zinc intake has even been reported in many developed countries like the United States. In fact, a latent zinc deficiency may affect as many as four million people in the U.S. When this deficiency affects older people, it constitutes a major risk factor because many of the elderly already have a compromised immune system from a lifetime of free radical damage and other causes, and so are particularly susceptible to infectious disease.

As with most minerals, when your body becomes deficient in zinc, it tries to fight back by excreting less of it, and absorbing more efficiently whatever zinc is present in the food eaten. But this is a short-lived attempt by the body to fight the deficiency. Human studies have shown that if you are zinc-deprived for six months or more the body's countermeasures do not persist.

DOSAGE

Many physicians may tell you that "you get plenty of zinc in your food, so you don't need to worry about it." However, this statement is not based on the current evidence, but on the fact that their medical-school curriculum was almost completely devoid of information on how to use nutrition to keep people healthy. And given what you now know about the importance of a healthy immune system, you should feel even more inclined to want to have adequate intakes of zinc.

When people consume diets low in zinc for an extended period of time, it appears that a zinc supplement of about eighty milligrams a day is more than adequate to restore zinc homeostasis in the body. However, unless you are significantly zinc-deficient, this is probably too high a supplemental dose; it may cause stomach indigestion. Based on my research, I decided to take *thirty milligrams of chelated zinc daily,* which is about double the government's recommended daily allowance for zinc in adults.

Zinc supplements are available just about anywhere. Chelated zinc, zinc methionine, and zinc sulphate are found in most stores that sell vitamin and mineral supplements, and they are effectively absorbed.

Fatty Acids and Phospholipids

Shielding cells from the ravaging effects of oxygen free radicals is one route to a long cellular Youthspan; maintaining and repairing cells after the free radicals that pierced that shield have done their inevitable dirty work is another.

The most understood way that free radicals damage cells is through attacks on the DNA, the cell proteins, and the cell membranes. Fatty acids and phospholipids are specific fatlike compounds that all of our cell membranes are composed of to a significant extent, and therefore they are needed in order for the cells to maintain and repair their cell membranes. That is because cell membranes are not stable entities; instead, they are constantly in a flux of discarding old parts and those damaged by free radicals and replacing them with new parts. Therefore, we need to keep them well supplied with the parts that they need, which include certain phospholipids and fatty acids.

There are other good reasons for maximizing our consumption of certain fatty acids and phospholipids. One reason is because Americans are consuming lots of "abnormal" fatty acids, called "trans"fatty acids, through high intakes of partially hydrogenated vegetable oils, such as those in margarine. Some scientists believe that when our cells go about their daily "upkeep and recycling" of their cell membranes, they may be using these transfatty acids in place of the natural fatty acids and phospholipids. It is not yet known what the long-term effects of this might be, but I personally don't want to give my cell membranes the wrong raw materials to keep themselves in top shape.

In addition, it has been shown that simply having low intakes of normal fatty acids and phospholipids in our diets is correlated with abnormal neurological function, including depression and decreased cognitive functions. A phospholipid called phosphatidylcholine (PPC) is very important in maintaining the integrity of the cell membranes of the liver cells that are involved in the daily detoxification of noxious substances we bring into our body, and fatty acids known as omega-3 fatty acids appear to provide several benefits to our bodies.

Phosphatidylcholine

WHAT IT IS AND HOW IT WORKS

Phosphatidylcholine (PPC) is a phospholipid that has been found to be especially useful in repairing and stabilizing the cell membranes of liver cells. Your body makes PPC, but it is very energy-demanding, and studies of people with existing liver disease suggest we don't make enough of it for maximal health of our liver cells.

Taking PPC is a particularly good idea if you drink alcohol, a major liver toxin. In fact, Dr. Charles Leiber, at the Mount Sinai School of Medicine in Manhattan, has shown that baboons consuming alcohol along with PPC supplements for several years were significantly less likely to progress to fibrosis and cirrhosis of the liver than those baboons drinking alcohol and not getting PPC.

A large number of human clinical trials, mostly in Europe, have tested PPC for years in people who already had some degree of liver damage, ranging from liver inflammation for various reasons to alcoholic fatty livers. Most of these studies revealed that patients who began taking PPC showed significant improvement in their liver-function tests. For example, a study at King's College in London, England, in 1982, on thirty people with chronic hepatitis-B infection (a viral infection of the liver) found that when half of these people received 2,300 milligrams of PPC daily for one year, along with their standard daily therapy for hepatitis B, they showed significant improvement in their liver structure (as revealed by biopsy) in comparison to the half who did not receive PPC. The PPC group also reported a significantly higher feeling of well-being than those people not receiving PPC. It is believed that PPC produces its benefits in the liver by stabilizing liver cell membranes, resulting in fewer liver cell enzymes leaking out into plasma, and less lipid peroxidation of liver cell membranes.

DOSAGE

People who have no known liver disease would seem to benefit from *500 to 1,000 milligrams of PPC daily*. I found the evidence regarding PPC and a healthy liver so compelling, along with its safety record, I now take *500 milligrams each day*.

The intakes of PPC that seem to be most effective in people

with existing liver damage range from about 1,000 milligrams to 4,500 milligrams (1.0 grams to 4.5 grams). No adverse effects have been seen at these doses. If you have existing liver disease, get a recent baseline of your liver-function tests from your physician. Start taking 1.5 grams of PPC daily for two months, and repeat your liver-function tests. If there is no significant improvement, take 3.0 grams daily for two months and test again. Do not take more than 4.0 grams daily.

Omega-3 Fatty Acids

WHAT THEY ARE AND HOW THEY WORK

Omega-3 fatty acids are a special type of polyunsaturated fatty acids that are found in both plants and animals. All our cell membranes contain lots of omega-3 fatty acids, particularly the cell membranes in our neurons. Therefore, as I described above, we need to keep our body supplied with these compounds if for no other reason than to keep our cell membranes supplied with the materials to constantly repair themselves.

The role of omega-3 fatty acids in enhancing Youthspan is basically twofold. First, several studies have shown that high intakes of omega-3 fatty acids seem to decrease the incidence of heart disease. This was first described in 1978, when John Dyerberg published a paper demonstrating that the fish that Eskimos consumed were very high in omega-3 fatty acids. He had begun this study because it was very puzzling that Eskimos had much lower rates of certain types of heart disease than people in the continental United States, despite the fact that their diets consisted almost exclusively of meat and fish.

Since then, several papers have suggested that omega-3 fatty acids decrease heart disease—but the question remains as to just how they do it. Several studies have shown they do it by blocking the synthesis of a special enzyme called thromboxane A2 (TAX). One of the jobs of TAX is to cause the small cells in our blood known as platelets to clump together whenever we cut ourselves. However, one of the reasons we get heart attacks and strokes is that TAX sometimes causes platelets to clump together when they shouldn't, and this clump of platelets then goes and clogs up our coronary arteries or an artery in our brain. Omega-3s seem to reduce the risk of this happening. Other strong evidence that has come out recently shows that omega-3s might decrease heart disease because they seem to prevent the development of what are called "arrhythmias" in our heart. Our hearts have a built-in electrical pacemaker, and sometimes it goes awry and sends our heart muscle into electrical pandemonium, which can cause sudden death. Omega-3s seem to help prevent this from happening.

Some scientists have questioned the benefits of omega-3 fatty acids in preventing heart disease, but a recent article in the respected medical journal *Lancet* has silenced most of them. This study looked at blood lipid profiles of fish eaters and vegetarians in two African populations, and found that the fish eaters (who were getting lots of omega-3s) fared much better with regard to heart disease than even the vegetarians. In fact, the multinational team concluded that ". . . the favorable risk factor profile originally described in Eskimos living on diets rich in omega-3 fatty acids is real and not overestimated."

The second important thing the omega-3 fatty acids seem to do for us is to stabilize the cell membrane of neurons, and this is believed to help prevent depression. Depression is the most commonly diagnosed mental disorder in the United States, and it has been increasing in North America in the last 100 years. Depression occurs mainly because certain neurotransmitters in the brain are released in inadequate amounts into the synapse. Because the part of the neuron's cell membrane that makes up the synapse is very high in omega-3 fatty acids, it is thought that a lack of these omega-3 fatty acids in the diet will then result in a lack of these fatty acids in these membranes; this in turn causes these synaptic membranes to fail to release their neurotransmitters properly, resulting in depression. In fact, a low consumption of omega-3 fatty acids during infancy or early childhood is believed to increase the chance of getting depression later in life. Rates of depression in North America are much higher than they are in Taiwan, Hong Kong, and Japan, where fish consumption is much higher.

Finally, ingestion of omega-3 fatty acids has been shown in recent years to both prevent and slow the growth of some human cancers such as colon, skin, and breast cancer in animals. For example, it was found that human cancer cells implanted into "nude" mice (mice with essentially no immune system) grew much more slowly in those mice consuming diets high in omega-3 fatty acids. Also, when nude mice were infected with human breast-cancer cells, those mice consuming higher levels of omega-3 fatty acids had a significantly reduced spread (metastasis) of the cancer to their lymph nodes and lungs.

DOSAGE

There are three omega-3 fatty acids which have shown the most importance for our long-term health: eicosapentaenoic acid (EPA), docosahexaenoic acid (DHA), and alpha linolenic acid (LA). We cannot make LA—it is therefore an *essential* fatty acid that must be supplied in our diet. Animals can make EPA and DHA from LA, but this process is extremely slow in humans, and we need to get EPA and DHA in our diets for the most part as well.

If you eat oily fish such as salmon, sardines, mackerel, or herring twice a week, you probably take in a sufficient amount of EPA and DHA. And if you eat lots of walnuts, soybeans, rapeseed, mustard greens, purslane, and spinach, you probably take in adequate amounts of LA. Flaxseed, or flaxmeal, and linseed oil from health food stores are other good, healthy sources of the omega-3 fatty acids, particularly LA.

But as always, the amounts of nutrients found in foods vary greatly, depending on where and when the food was grown and how it has been processed. In addition, eating oily fish can supply you with lots of unwanted fat. A recommended daily allowance for omega-3s has not been firmly established. However, a healthy intake has been shown to be around *300 milligrams daily of LA, and 100 to 200 milligrams daily of EPA and DHA.*

If you do not buy them separately, but instead buy capsules that contain fish oil (which has a mix of mostly EPA and DHA), do not buy more than a month's supply at a time, and keep the bottle in the refrigerator to prevent rancidity. If you take fish-oil capsules, you should buy flaxmeal and add a few tablespoons to your food every evening, to make sure you are getting enough LA as well.

Note: A recent study suggests that if you have an autoimmune disorder, taking about 900 milligrams of EPA and 600 to 700 milligrams of DHA daily can be very helpful in alleviating its symptoms.

Antiinflammatories

Aspirin/NSAIDs

WHAT THEY ARE AND HOW THEY WORK

Aspirin, or acetylsalicylic acid, is one of the oldest medications in use today; it is still the most commonly found substance in most medicine cabinets. Its active ingredient is found in the bark of the willow tree as well as in oil of wintergreen. Aspirin's best-known use is as an antiinflammatory, countering inflammations that cause body aches and pains. But recent evidence demonstrates that those little white pills have miraculous disease-preventing qualities, particularly regarding the three most dreaded geriatric diseases: cardiovascular disease (heart disease and stroke), cancer, and dementia.

The way aspirin reduces inflammation is by blocking an enzyme our bodies needs to make a group of compounds that promote inflammation and its symptoms. For some time many researchers have felt that chronic, long-term inflammation is an important part of a series of events that leads to many types of cancers. Therefore, aspirin as well as other antiinflammatory drugs (such as ibuprofen) have been studied in this regard, producing growing evidence that they significantly reduce the incidence of many types of cancer in laboratory animals. More importantly, recent human studies show that people who use aspirin regularly develop significantly less colorectal cancer than people who do not. Currently, a number of large human clinical trials are underway to determine if other human cancers are inhibited by regular use of aspirin.

Aspirin already has a growing mainstream reputation for preventing platelet aggregation and clumping in our blood. A whole shelf-full of studies has shown that if people who have suffered one heart attack or stroke are given a small amount of aspirin daily, their risk of a second heart attack or stroke goes down dramatically. For example, by the late 1980s, twenty-five human trials involving antiplatelet aggregation therapy (using mostly aspirin) had been completed in a total of about 29,000 people who had already had a heart attack or stroke. In 1988, the worldwide Antiplatelet Trialists' Collabortion (ATC) conducted a statistical overview of all of these twenty-five research trials. This ATC study found that those people taking aspirin or other anticlotting compounds regularly had a much lower incidence of having a second heart attack or stroke, when compared to those people who had previously had a stroke or heart attack, but were not taking antiplatelet compounds.

Now evidence convincingly shows that using aspirin to prevent a first heart attack is a good idea as well. The U.S. Physicians Health Study involved over 22,000 physicians, half of whom took one aspirin tablet every other day, the other half a placebo every other day. The placebo part of this study was terminated after five years because analysis of the data showed that the doctors taking aspirin were having heart attacks 44 percent less frequently than those physicians who were taking the placebo. They terminated the study so that the doctors taking the placebo could start taking an aspirin every other day themselves. Several large clinical trials looking at aspirin usage and risk of heart disease and stroke are currently under way.

There is also a growing literature that suggests chronic inflammation in the brain may play a large role in both the onset and progression of Alzheimer's disease. For example, it's been found in several recent studies that people using over-the-counter antiinflammatory drugs called NSAIDs (non-steroidal antiinflammatory drugs—examples are Nuprin, Aleve, Motrin, and Clinoril) and/or aspirin moderately over several years for various aches and pains had a much lower likelihood of acquiring Alzheimer's disease than people who did not.

DOSAGE

The effective dose of aspirin to prevent a heart attack or stroke appears to range from *75 to about 325 milligrams a day* (one adult aspirin tablet is 325 milligrams), or one adult tablet every other day. One aspirin a day (or every other day) is also a reasonable dose to help lower your risk of Alzheimer's disease and colon cancer.

But it is important to note that taking more than one aspirin a day does not increase your protection and can possibly harm you. This is because aspirin can cause stomach and intestinal ulcers, which can lead to serious bleeding. If you have, or suspect you have existing ulcers you need to consult your physician before starting to take aspirin regularly.

In the several studies which showed that the people who reported regularly using some type of NSAID were much less likely to get Alzheimer's disease, the dosage used varied considerably among the study participants. My advice is that if you now use any NSAIDs at all on a fairly regular basis for some condition, keep using them as needed; and if you are using them as a preventative, do not take more than one pill daily

Note I: acetaminophen (Tylenol) did not seem to provide any protection in any of the studies where it was used, so I cannot recommend it for preventative therapy.

Note II: If you are taking any type of blood-thinning medication, such as Warfarin, be absolutely sure to check with your doctor before taking any aspirin or NSAID.

CHAPTER NINE

Basic Mega-Chicken Soup Tools II: Stress-Reduction Techniques

What They Are and How They Work

*B*oth physical and mental stress can initiate a chain of neurological events that result in the release of excessive catecholamines and cortisol into the blood. These two hormones are responsible for much of the stress-induced damage in our bodies, including the brain. Even our bones suffer, as chronically high levels of stress hormone dismantle healthy bone and cause fractures. Stress can also exacerbate an existing disease from another cause and make you even sicker, which in turn increases stress even more. So stress reduction will not only enable you to avoid these problems, it will also pay off in more functional immune and gastrointestinal systems, a healthier cardiovascular system, and increased fertility. Thus, it is one of the keys to a Youthspan-friendly lifestyle.

The idea behind stress-reduction or relaxation therapy is to calm a hyperactive sympathetic nervous system and hypothalamo-pituitary-adrenal axis, thus decreasing the release of the neurotransmitters and hormones that cause stress-related problems. Many techniques have been found effective in this regard, including biofeedback, meditation, and guided imagery. The so-called relaxation response that occurs in different forms with each of these stress-reduction strategies has primarily been applied to the treatment of cardiovascular disease, particularly through blood pressure reduction—Dr. Dean Ornish, a clinical professor of medicine at the University of California at San Francisco, has actually been able to reverse the blockage cf coronary arteries by employing a combination of meditation and other stress-reduction exercises, moderate physical exercise, and a vegetarian diet. In fact, these measures can have positive effects on all of your body's systems.

Below are some psychological exercises that you can utilize very effectively to help manage your stress. Later on, I'll show how physical exercise can also reduce stress.

Biofeedback

WHAT IT IS AND HOW IT WORKS

Before the 1960s, most scientists believed that such things as heart rate, blood pressure, digestion, and muscle behavior could not be controlled by an individual without the help of drugs, claims to the contrary by yoga adepts notwithstanding. Now biofeedback used in conjunction with techniques such as meditation, progressive relaxation, and guided imagery, is widely accepted by most of the medical community. Basically, biofeedback is a setup for "teaching" your body how to control its responses. The "feedback" is information on the how the body is currently responding, which is then fed back to the individual via a simple signal, usually a sound or a flashing light. So, for example, if your aim is to lower your blood pressure by self-induced relaxation, the feedback device will tell you when your blood pressure starts to drop.

Other kinds of information these devices can gather and feed back include skin temperature, and skin electrical conductivity (galvanic skin response, also used in "lie detectors"), with low skin temperatures and electrical conductivity indicative of deepening relaxation. Still other indicators of decreased stress responses are a lessening of muscle tension (which can be monitored with an electromyogram), lowered heart rate (measured by monitoring pulse rate), and particular types of brain waves (measured with an electroencephalogram) that are seen when we are relaxed. Eventually, a person can learn how to regulate the parameter in question (heart rate, muscle tension, brain waves, and so on) in a stress-reducing direction without the aid of the biofeedback device. Biofeedback has been used successfully to treat several stress-related disorders, including insomnia, migraine headaches, temporomandibular-joint syndrome, and gastrointestinal disorders.

HOW TO DO IT

Although you can now buy biofeedback devices in some health food stores and catalogs, I think your best bet is to start this technique with the help of an experienced professional. Such professionals are fairly easy to find; many clinical psychologists are trained in this technique. To find names and phone numbers of practitioners of biofeedback in your state, call the Association for Applied Psychophysiology and Biofeedback, in Wheat Ridge, Colorado, at (303) 422-8436. You can also get information on biofeedback practitioners from the Biofeedback Certification Institute of America by calling (303) 420-2902.

Meditation

WHAT IT IS AND HOW IT WORKS

During the 1960s reports reached the West that yoga meditation masters in India could perform extraordinary feats of bodily control and altered states of consciousness. For psychologists and practitioners of mind-body medicine, this technique offered the promise of being a way we could voluntarily control our "involuntary" nervous system—particularly the sympathetic nervous system which, as you have seen, becomes dangerously hyperactive during stress.

There are two basic categories of meditation: concentrative and mindful. In the former, the practitioner focuses on her breath, an image, or a sound, like a mantra—the focus in transcendental meditation. Mindfulness meditation, according to Dr. Joan Borysenko, a pioneer in mind/body medicine, "involves becoming aware of the continuously passing parade of sensations, feelings, images, thoughts, sounds, smells, and so forth, without becoming involved with habitual worries or images." Both approaches allow the person to achieve a calm, nonreactive, stress-reduced state of mind. Perhaps the best studied of the Western-adopted meditation techniques is Vedic yoga, Maharishi Mahesh Yogi's transcendental meditation, currently practiced by an estimated four million people. Clinical studies have shown that a regular practice of TM can produce reduced heart and respiratory rates, and also reduce plasma cortisol.

HOW TO DO IT

The basic idea behind yogic meditation is to empty the mind for an extended period of time by narrowing its focus to one object: a single image, like the flame of a candle, or a single imagined sound, like a mantra. With the mind focused on this one object, all other thoughts and concerns gradually drop away. For ten to thirty minutes (or more), you can achieve a relaxed but conscious state that has profound effects, both psychologically and physically. Indeed, the physical effects can be measured in changes of brain waves and, over time, by markers of oxidative stress.

I can personally recommend transcendental meditation as an effective and easily learned form of meditation. These days, there are instructors in this technique available in almost every American city (I will give you some help finding them below). Other meditation techniques can be learned from yoga teachers who also can be found in most cities.

For the do-it-yourselfers among you, I offer the following two techniques.

Meditation Exercise I

SERENE MIND

A. Sit comfortably on a cushion or chair with your hips higher than your knees, your back straight, and your hands resting on your knees, palms facing up.

B. Choose a point three or four feet ahead of you on the floor and fix your eyes on it. Keep your eyes on that spot. (Blinking is okay.)

C. Breathing deeply and regularly, remain in this position for ten to thirty minutes. If you become aware of any tension in your chest or shoulders, breathe into these areas, relaxing them.

D. Listen to the sound of your own breathing. Allow any thoughts that enter your mind to gently drift away—but do not actively push them away.

Meditation Exercise II

MANTRA

A. Seated as above, but with your eyes closed, silently repeat a mantra in your mind. Some people find special affinities for certain mantras like *Om Shanti* and *So* (on inhalation), *Hum* (on exhale). But Harvard psychologist Robert Benson, author of *The Relaxation Response,* believes any single- or double-syllable word will do the trick. So I suggest the mantra, *Young-er.*

B. Continue repeating the mantra in steady rhythm for ten to thirty minutes.

C. Allow any thoughts that enter your mind to gently drift away— but do not actively push them away.

Resources

The Institute of Transpersonal Psychology in Stanford, California, is a source of information about meditation research and teachers, and can be reached at (414) 327-2066. The Mind-Body Clinic at the New Deaconess Hospital, a division of Harvard Medical School, can teach you how to relax and get rid of your stress. Call them at (617) 632-9530. For those interested in where you can learn TM, call the Maharishi International University in Fairfield, Iowa, at (515) 472-5031, and they will provide you with information on where to learn transcendental meditation.

🍂

Part V

FLAB INTO MUSCLE, SLOTH INTO ENERGY

*S*trength and energy are the basic stuff of youth; we dread losing them in our later years. And so the Youthspan Program's most *powerfully felt* effect on us is our increased muscle power and higher level of stamina. That a combination of hormone replacement therapy, vitamin supplements, diet, and exercise can deliver this basic stuff of youth to us in our forties, fifties, sixties, and seventies feels like nothing short of a miracle.

Objective results in this area are easily measured by looking at the bathroom scale and in the mirror, by gauging how much more weight we can lift, and how much longer we can walk or play tennis or simply go without rest. If we want more quantifiable results, we can map our progress on a computerized treadmill that measures how many calories we burn, how fast we burn them, and for how long. Yet for most of us, the most satisfying objective results are the appraising comments of friends—"My God, you look as fit as a twenty-year-old!"

But turning flab into muscle is much more than a cosmetic transition—although it is most certainly that too. Greater body strength, along with less dead weight to carry around, translates into greater mobility, and a greater range of activities available to us—from sports to outdoor work. Indeed, having the energy to use and develop muscles has the trickle-down effect of giving us better overall control of our bodies, including better balance—literally, better poise. And, of course, there is the sheer pleasure of athleticism. Similarly, more accessible and sustainable energy translates into more waking hours in each day, as well as a broader range of available activities—both work tasks and recreation that require abiding energy to perform.

REVERSING THAT "CAN'T DO" ATTITUDE

Aging is often characterized by a "Can't Do" attitude: "Can't do that, it'll tire me out," or "Forget about doing that, it'll give me a heart attack." This attitude, of course, becomes self-fulfilling and self-perpetuating.

But here again is a place where you can reverse the cycle and get it spiraling upward. If you take the supplements, engage the diet, and do the exercises I recommend here, you will very quickly discover untapped reservoirs of energy that cannot be denied— you simply have to do something with all that new-found vigor. And pretty soon, instead of saying, "Can't do that," you find your- self saying, "Let me at it—whatever it is!"

This is not merely a change in self-esteem or mood (although hormone supplements and endorphin-producing physical exercise can substantially boost mood on their own), it is a complete change in life philosophy and personal expectations. People with low energy and a limited range of possible activities retreat from life, usually in the direction of the couch, while people with high energy and a large variety of endeavors to choose from embrace life. Life *is* energy. The more energy you have, the more life you have.

YOU'RE NEVER TOO OLD TO FEEL YOUNG

Much of what we consider normal aging has nothing to do with aging *per se,* only with lack of muscle use, which leads to muscle atrophy and disability. So when an older person takes up a supervised graduated exercise program—especially along with the benefits of hormone replacement and a nutritious diet—he may very well reverse many of the so-called normal symptoms of aging. He will be able to rise out of a chair or get out of a car much more easily, stand straighter, walk more briskly and for a longer period of time, dance, play—you name it.

When it comes to relatively swift and dramatic results, hormone-replacement therapy* is pretty much in a category of its own. And there is a synergy of hormone replacement with diet and exercise that has an added bonus: each element motivates us to seek out whatever else can help us become slimmer, stronger, and more energetic.

---

*I have somewhat arbitrarily divided my discussion of hormones between this and a forthcoming section, "Feeling Young and Sexy" (Chapters 13 and 14). Here, we will look into DHEA, melatonin, and growth-hormone replacement; later we will look into estrogen and testosterone replacement.

CHAPTER TEN

Muscle and Energy Tools I: Hormones

*N*othing has fueled the Youthspan Revolution as much as recent studies involving various types of hormone-replacement therapy. We happen to be living at the happy moment when the ability of certain hormones to preserve youth has been definitively established in animal studies, and studies of these same hormones in humans have begun in earnest and appear very promising. The hormones that have shown the most promise at this stage of the research, with respect to having great potential for increasing our Youthspan, are the protein hormone *growth hormone* (GH), the indole hormone *melatonin,* and a diverse group of steroid hormones, namely the *estrogens* (the most important one being estradiol), and the androgens (*DHEA and testosterone*).

All of these hormones have been shown to decline with age in most mammals (including humans), and many studies have shown that these declines correlate very well with the onset of many diseases and other problems associated with aging. DHEA, melatonin, and GH seem to decline in both men and women as we age. Testosterone clearly declines with age in men, and some studies are now suggesting that postmenopausal women, too, suffer effects from a loss of testosterone. Estrogen decline seems to only occur in postmenopausal women and not older men (whose estrogen levels may actually go up). Estrogen is the only hormone that has already been used for decades in the prevention of disease; the others are relative newcomers to the prevention scene, although GH has been used for years to treat dwarfism in children.

It is certainly well known that hormones regulate many important body functions, so a reduction of them as we age implies a loss in normal regulation of these functions. Conversely, it seems logical that resupplementing these hormones, to maintain the levels normally present in a young person well into his or her middle age, keeps these body functions performing vigorously. The idea is that a fifty-year-old body with a functional blood hormone level of a twenty-five-year-old is a body that feels and behaves in many critical ways as if it *is* twenty-five.

A clue to why hormones figure so prominently in youth maintenance is found in the fact that many of them are involved in reproduction when we are young (particularly testosterone and estrogen, but also GH, melatonin, and DHEA). Many population geneticists will tell you that life spans within a species have evolved to optimize reproductive schedules, which natural selection has operated on through at least two biological determinants which also affect total lifespan: 1) the age at which a species first becomes capable of reproducing itself; and 2) the mortality rate after the first successful reproduction. Taken together, these observations suggest that evolution has provided for each species to live long enough to reproduce sufficient offspring, and to take care of its progeny; then, assuming its life-insurance premiums are paid up, it is free to die. In other words, biological aging accelerates after one's body senses it has outlasted its reproductive usefulness. In fact, comparative studies between mammalian species show that the earlier in life that a species is capable of reproducing, the shorter its overall lifespan will be. Now, all of this implies that our reproductive hormones may be partly responsible for keeping us young, that when the hormones begin to decline after our reproductive "peak," our bodies begin to decline as well. This would certainly offer credence to the idea of replacing these hormones.

Women have been taking estrogen supplementation after menopause since the 1950s, with excellent results. In fact, it is surprising that it took another thirty-odd years before anyone made the cognitive jump from replacing that hormone to replacing other hormones that decline with age. One reason is that many hormones were not synthetically available until fairly recently, and that their only source would have been from cadavers, which would have been expensive to harvest.

Currently, only DHEA and melatonin are available without a physician's prescription. Again, keep in mind that only a small percentage of physicians are staying abreast of the significant medical research that shows an emerging role for hormone-replacement therapy in preventing, as well as reversing, many age-associated problems. So you need to go into the doctor's office with as much knowledge as possible if you are going to try to use any of these hormones. I am inundated with questions about the potential youth-enhancing effects of these substances, not only by former medical students who are now practicing medicine (because they, in turn, are being inundated by questions from *their* patients), but also by friends who are interested in these substances, and want to show their doctor where to find the clinical information that is available about them.

Now, here is something that may surprise you—coming as it does from a scientist who feels strongly that people should take charge of their own health—with the exception of melatonin, I do not believe anyone should take any of these hormones without the supervision of a physician. That is because the potential side effects of most of these hormones are significant if used improperly. I have been hearing stories about young men taking handfuls of DHEA because they heard that it can be converted to testosterone and, therefore, they think, will make them more muscular; there is absolutely no evidence that this is true. But what is true is that these young men run a sizable risk of developing liver problems, and eventual prostate cancer, not to mention uncontrollable outbursts of aggressive behavior.

Baseline Hormone Levels

But again, finding the right doctor may not be easy, because not every doctor agrees that a decline of DHEA, testosterone, estrogen, and growth hormone to levels well below those of a twenty-five-year-old presents a genuine threat to your Youthspan, and therefore should be treated. On the contrary, the majority of American physicians will only conclude that you have a deficiency if your hormone levels are significantly below the average for *someone your age*. What this means, of course, is that most physicians *accept aging as normal*.

But even when you do find a physician who understands the benefits of restoring certain hormones to their youthful levels, he cannot operate under precise conditions if he does not know what your *personal* hormone levels were in your late twenties or early thirties. This is not an awful state of affairs, but it is a less than ideal way to determine how much of a particular hormone you should be taking. So, if you are presently in your twenties or thirties, I strongly suggest that you get your plasma-hormone levels measured now and do so once every two to three years. This will allow you to have accurate target hormone levels to shoot for when you are older and in need of supplementation; it will also accurately measure the rate of decline of your plasma hormones over the years. If you can, you should have your blood samples drawn each time at the same laboratory or office, and at the same hour of the day, under fasting conditions, to minimize sample-to-sample variation. Ideally, young men should get baseline blood measurements of DHEA, DHEAS (sulphated DHEA), and insulin-like growth factor 1 (IGF-1, one of many IGFs which carry out most of the effects of growth hormone). They also should have an androgen profile done (testosterone, dihydrotestosterone, and androstenedione). And finally, get what is called a GH provocation test (a test that involves giving you a compound that provokes the release of GH from your pituitary, to evaluate how responsive your pituitary is to such a stimulus). Baseline information on plasma melatonin in the second or third decade of life may also be helpful.

Women in their twenties or thirties should have their blood DHEA, DHEAS, and IGF-1 measured also, and should repeat these measurements every two or three years. Baseline levels of the steroid hormones are less useful in premenopausal women because these hormones vary greatly throughout the menstrual cycle, and can even vary considerably from one cycle to the next.

Here, then, is a description of the potential benefits of DHEA,

GH, and melatonin replacement. I have deferred information about EHRT and testosterone to the next section.

DHEA

WHAT IT IS AND HOW IT WORKS

Dehydroepiandrosterone (DHEA) is a steroid hormone and a weak androgen. It is made predominantly in our adrenal cortex, but a small amount is also produced in our gonads (ovaries and testicles). DHEA is made by our adrenal glands primarily during the morning hours, and levels decline considerably over the course of the day. The daily production of DHEA by our adrenals peaks at between twenty-five to thirty years of age, and declines steadily after that point (about a 2 percent drop each year). By the time we are ninety years old, we normally have less than 5 percent of the DHEA concentration in our blood that we had when we were twenty-five.

One of the more commonly reported effects by people taking DHEA is an almost immediate boost in energy and feelings of well-being. In fact, one of the first studies of DHEA in humans was done by the Department of Reproductive Medicine at the University of California Medical School in San Diego, and reported in 1995. The authors stated that after taking fifty milligrams of DHEA each evening for just a few weeks, both the men and women in this study reported a "remarkable increase in perceived physical and psychological well-being."

But elevated energy and mood are just the tip of the iceberg in terms of DHEA's youth-enhancing effects. DHEA definitely causes improvements in different types of cognitive function in animals, and now several studies have begun to show that DHEA effectively improves certain types of memory in aging humans, as well. A study by Dr. Owen Wokowitz from the University of California at San Francisco found that elevating the plasma-DHEA levels in clinically depressed patients to the levels of young people produced significant improvements in both memory and mood. It has also been found that a single oral dose of DHEA given to volunteers produced a significant increase in REM sleep in these individuals. This is important, because REM sleep has been associated with memory storage.

Declining DHEA levels have been correlated with an increased risk for heart disease. Part of the reason for this may be insulin, the hormone made by the pancreas, which promotes the uptake of the major blood sugar (glucose) out of the blood and into cells where it can be used as a source of energy. Millions of Americans who become overweight when they reach their forties and fifties acquire Type-II diabetes, and the many chronic problems associated with it, as a result of the persistently high blood levels of both glucose and insulin seen in this disorder. That's because it is now well known that both glucose and insulin can actually harm many of our tissues, if they remain chronically elevated.

William Regelson, an oncologist at the Medical College of Virginia, and the author of an excellent book on DHEA and other hormones (*The Superhormone Promise*), believes that DHEA acts as a buffer for the negative effects of consistently high levels of insulin in our blood vessels. In fact, his colleague, Dr. John Nestler, believes that the gradual increase in plasma-insulin levels that occur in many of us as we age may be at least partly responsible for the gradual simultaneous decrease in plasma DHEA. In one study, Nestler treated men having high insulin levels with drugs to bring the levels down; when the levels dropped, their plasma-DHEA levels rose markedly, reinforcing Nestler's theory that high blood levels of insulin may suppress blood-DHEA levels. DHEA may ultimately prove to be an effective treatment for preventing many of the serious problems associated with Type-II diabetes, which are secondary to high insulin levels.

DHEA produces other effects which lower our risk of heart disease as well. One of these is its ability to prevent platelets from clotting abnormally, thus reducing the likelihood of a clot lodging in a narrow blood vessel and cutting off the blood supply to critical organs, including the heart. Furthermore, DHEA has been shown to lower the levels of LDL, which is also associated with an increased risk of cardiovascular disease.

As we have seen, many of our immune-system functions naturally decline with age, but in animal studies, DHEA has reduced this decline by modifying certain types of cytokines, special hormones that control the immune system. Another way DHEA may enhance immunity could be through its modulation of cortisol, the major stress hormone. In animal studies, DHEA seems to "temper" cortisol's effects. For example, animals that are given DHEA and then put into controlled, stressful situations, tend to suffer much less disease as a result of this stress compared to animals put in the same stressful conditions that do not receive DHEA.

More recent studies have shown that DHEA has important effects on the human immune system as well. For example, when nine healthy men averaging sixty-four years of age took DHEA nightly for about five months, the DHEA significantly elevated their circulating levels of natural killer cells. A natural killer cell is a type of lymphocyte that is important for our immune system to detect cancer cells.

Another study of elderly men reported in 1997, showed that those men taking oral DHEA each night had a significant increase in a number of vital immune parameters. This study also found that men taking DHEA experienced significant increases in their insulin-like growth factor-1 levels. (See section below on growth hormone.) In addition, a report appearing in the *Annals of the New York Academy of Science* followed a group of individuals over the age of sixty-five who were vaccinated against the influenza virus. Some of these individuals were given DHEA for two consecutive days beginning the day they were vaccinated, while the rest got a placebo. The group receiving DHEA had *a four-fold greater antibody response to the vaccine*. This is very promising news, because one of the problems with vaccinating older people is that they often do not generate enough antibodies to the vaccine for it to be effective, due to their age-weakened immune systems.

Also, in the first study of its kind, a report from San Francisco General Hospital demonstrated that low levels of plasma DHEA predicted which HIV-positive patients were most likely to progress to full-blown AIDS. A later study of HIV-positive patients done at Louisiana State University evaluated the blood levels of plasma DHEAS and "helper T-cells" (the important immune cells which are destroyed by the AIDS virus), and also found that those who had the lowest DHEAS blood levels predictably had the lowest helper T-cell levels in their blood. What this suggests is that DHEA may somehow keep the HIV virus in check, although this has not been proven conclusively.

Additional clinical trials are currently underway to more fully determine what role DHEA might have in treating diseases directly involving the immune system. Some of these have produced results on the relationship of DHEA to autoimmune diseases like systemic lupus erythematosus (SLE). One study followed ten female SLE patients using DHEA daily for six months; at the end of this time, several symptoms of SLE were improved in these women, and they were able to get along with less of their immune-suppressing drugs.

DOSAGE

For starters, most people under the age of fifty should probably *not* be using DHEA, as they are presumably still producing sufficient amounts of it to ward off most of the problems associated with its deficiency. *But most people over age fifty should seriously consider starting on DHEA supplements.*

None of the methods that follow are as easy as just grabbing some pills off the shelf and chucking them down your throat every morning. But the Youthspan benefits of taking DHEA in safe, correct amounts is well worth the trouble of doing it properly.

Men over fifty: Before starting on a DHEA regime, have a complete physical exam, including a complete blood chemistry, digital prostate exam, and a plasma prostate specific antigen (PSA) determination. Then, have your serum DHEA, DHEAS, testosterone (total and "free" levels), androstenedione, and estradiol levels quantified. Have your blood drawn in the morning before eating each time you measure these hormones, as their levels normally fluctuate throughout the day.

Assuming you have no health problems, and that your hormone tests show your plasma DHEA and DHEAS levels are low compared to the levels seen in youthful men (which they almost certainly will be), the next step is to start taking *25 milligrams of DHEA each morning* when our adrenal glands normally make the most of it. Also, you should eat some food with your DHEA to facilitate its absorption from your intestine.

After three months, have your blood drawn again in the morning before eating by the same laboratory that did your baseline tests. (Do not take your DHEA supplement on the morning you have your blood drawn.) Now compare these new DHEA and DHEAS levels with your baseline levels to see how much they have increased. Although these are only averages, youthful levels of plasma DHEA have been shown to be in the range of ten to twenty nanomoles per liter of plasma (nMol/L) for healthy males, with DHEA levels in young healthy females being approximately one-third lower than those seen in young males; youthful levels of DHEAS average from 6,000 to 10,000 nMol/L in both males and females. If your DHEA and DHEAS levels have not increased to this range after three months of use, you should consider increasing your dosage, starting with an increase to fifty milligrams. But first you need to check if there have been any large changes in the hormones that DHEA can be converted to (i.e., testosterone, androstenedione, and estrogen). You should actually consider cutting back your morning DHEA dosage if any of the other measured hormones have increased dramatically above their baseline levels. Finally, you and your doctor also need to consider if there has been any significant change in your hematocrit, your plasma PSA levels, or your prostate size, or if you are experiencing any adverse side effects from your current DHEA dosage.

If your serum DHEA has *increased* well above the average levels for males in their twenties, you should cut back to fifteen milligrams of DHEA in the morning. (There is no evidence that DHEA levels higher than the physiological ranges seen in youth are beneficial; indeed, they may be harmful.)

Whether it is determined you need to increase, cut back, or maintain your current DHEA dosage, you need to retest your blood hormone levels again in three months and reevaluate them. Once you get your hormone levels in a safe and youthful range with no side effects, then it is advisable to do the above testing only on a yearly basis.

Postmenopausal Women: I do not believe women still having regular menstrual cycles should be using DHEA. These women make more estrogen than postmenopausal women, and since DHEA can easily be converted to estrogen in some women, this could result in dangerously high levels of estrogen in their bodies, particularly at certain stages of the menstrual cycle. In addition, since DHEA can be made into different types of estrogens, as well as androgens like testosterone, using DHEA may produce abnormal menstrual cycles in young women. Since menopause tends to occur at around the same time that a woman's DHEA levels are becoming significantly lower anyway (in her early fifties), this seems like a logical time to institute this therapy.

In general, the procedure for taking DHEA is essentially the same for these women as it is for men, *starting with 25 milligrams in the morning* and taking it from there. (Obviously women do not need a PSA or prostate digital exam.) However, women should get a complete blood chemistry before starting DHEA, and it would be a good idea for the women considering taking this supplement to have a baseline mammogram after age forty-five, and to get one every two years until age fifty or so, and then one every year.

Also, just like men, women need to have pre-DHEA/DHEAS blood work done, and post-DHEA/DHEAS blood work done every few months after beginning to take DHEA supplements, until a new, more youthful blood-DHEA/DHEAS level is firmly established. Furthermore, a postmenopausal woman who decides to take DHEA needs to take into account whether she is also taking estrogen hormone-replacement therapy (EHRT) before beginning to use DHEA. (See Chapter 13 for information on EHRT.) As DHEA can be converted to estrogen, using it might increase blood estrogen levels into an unsafe range.

But there is a flip side to this logic as well. Postmenopausal women who want to use EHRT, but who are hesitant to use the "horse-urine estrogens" that are currently the most commonly prescribed, could get a dual benefit from the use of DHEA because it may also increase serum-estrogen levels, providing "natural" estrogen during the menopause. This could either allow you to have all the benefits of EHRT without having to take any synthetic, unnatural estrogens or at the least could result in you having to take far less of the synthetic estrogens.

There will also be some women who convert significant amounts of their DHEA supplement to testosterone. This may be beneficial or adverse. For example, some studies have now shown that in many postmenopausal women testosterone levels that decline along with estrogen levels are responsible for the loss of libido often experienced by these women, even those taking EHRT. For this reason, some physicians now include testosterone along with estrogen for their postmenopausal patients using EHRT.

However, while some extra testosterone can be beneficial, having too much of it can cause excessive hair growth (hirsutism), an increased hematocrit, or can potentially block the beneficial effects of supplemental estrogen. You will certainly know if you grow ex-cess hair—and you should be getting blood work done every few months for the first year after starting DHEA to determine changes in your hematocrit. You will also know if any excess testosterone you produce prevents your estrogen from working, because suddenly you will develop some of the subjective symptoms of estrogen-deficiency—like hot flashes, vaginal dryness, and irritability—that had previously vanished when you started taking EHRT. If any of these things happen, you need to work with your physician on cutting back on your DHEA supplementation. Or you and your doctor can consider changing your method of taking DHEA, or the form of DHEA you are using.

FORMS OF DHEA

DHEA is now available in capsule, pill, or cream. Most DHEA you see in stores is in pill form, usually ten, twenty-five, or fifty milli-grams. Your doctor can order DHEA from a compounding pharmacy in any dosage or form for you, even in lozenges or ointments. One of the newest forms of DHEA is called "micronized" DHEA. Nor-mally, DHEA taken orally is absorbed from your intestine and goes directly to your liver in what are known as the hepatic-portal blood vessels, where some of it is metabolized before it even gets into your general circulation—and it is this "first pass" through the liver that results in the conversion of large amounts of DHEA to testoster-one in many people. Micronized DHEA taken orally is thought to mostly bypass the liver, being carried away from the intestine by the lymphatic system instead of the hepatic-portal blood vessels. Both men and women enjoy more efficient absorption of DHEA by taking this form of it. It was also believed that bypassing the liver might minimize the conversion of DHEA to testosterone in some women. However, a 1996 study showed that micronized DHEA taken orally increased blood-testosterone levels along with blood-DHEA levels in women. On the other hand, DHEA cream adminis-tered vaginally increased DHEA levels, but not testosterone levels. Therefore, vaginal administration of DHEA might be an option for postmenopausal women wanting an increased plasma DHEA level, but not an increased testosterone level.

Currently, almost all of the forms of DHEA you buy in stores is produced by extracting a sterol called diosgenin from wild yams.

The diosgenin is then subjected to some chemical reactions in the laboratory, producing DHEA. Your body cannot produce these chemical reactions which convert diosgenin to DHEA. Therefore, do not be fooled by products which are called "DHEA Precursors," "Natural DHEA" from wild yams, or "Wild Yam Extract." These products are *not* DHEA.

Growth Hormone

WHAT IT IS AND HOW IT WORKS

Growth hormone (GH) is best known for its role in regulating physical growth. In fact, until the last decade, its only clinical use was for treatment of GH-deficient children who would otherwise suffer from dwarfism. (GH has been available to treat these children since the late 1950s, but the only source was pituitary glands taken from human cadavers, so the supply was restricted. In 1987, a synthetic form of GH was approved by the FDA.) But now it has become clear that GH plays an important role in fully grown adults—a role that has a major impact on Youthspan. This impact is seen in our muscle/fat ratio, the health and vigor of critical organs, and the appearance and resilience of our skin.

While most of us have plenty of GH during our younger years, almost all adults experience a decline in the amount of GH that is released as we age; after around age thirty, GH concentrations in blood drop about 14 percent for every decade of life, which results in a drop in the levels of the IGFs as well. During this same period, our body composition changes with a progressive decline in lean body mass (muscle) and a progressive increase in the amount of fat we store. So even if there is not a large change in total weight, we are made of a lot less muscle and a lot more fat as we creep along. Our organs, such as the brain, liver, and kidneys, also start to shrink as we age. The net effect of these losses includes many of the infirmities associated with age, particularly general fatigue, declining energy, and lost mobility and strength.

The late Dr. Daniel Rudman, of the University of Wisconsin, first suggested in 1985 that GH supplementation might reverse these negative changes in body composition that start to occur after age thirty. He experimented with synthetic GH injections on twenty-one late-middle-aged men who all had the classic symptoms of age-related loss of lean body mass and increase in fat. And lo and behold, he found that six months after starting treatments, these men gained an average of 9 percent lean body mass, with a 14 percent loss in fat—all without any change in their regular diet or exercise patterns! As an unexpected bonus, their skin became thicker, with fewer wrinkles.

In a follow-up study, men between the ages of sixty and eighty received GH injections over a one-year period; their lean body mass increased 6 percent, their body fat declined 15 percent, their skin thickness increased 4 percent, and their muscle increased 11 percent. The controls in this study, who did not receive GH, simply continued to "normally" decline with age, losing an additional 4 percent of their lean body mass and 6 percent of their skin thickness. This powerful evidence has now been replicated in several studies involving both women and men.

Some of these studies have shown that in addition to the above benefits, GH supplementation can produce improvements in our cardiovascular functions, in part because GH decreases the levels of LDL. There is also growing evidence that maintaining youthful levels of GH helps keep the aging immune system in tip-top condition.

A large protein hormone manufactured in our anterior pituitary gland, GH's release is controlled by other hormones coming from the hypothalamus, a brain structure that sits above the anterior pituitary gland. Like most anterior pituitary hormones, GH is released in pulses into the blood rather than continuously secreted; the amount and frequency of these pulses are important in the effectiveness of the hormone. Like most protein hormones, GH works by traveling to different sites in the body and binding to a receptor. Once a pulse of GH is released into the blood from the anterior pituitary gland, one of the first things it does is to go to the liver and bind its receptor, which then stimulates the synthesis of several different IGFs. In fact, it appears that it is these IGFs that produce most of the beneficial effects ascribed to GH.

DOSAGE

In 1996, the FDA approved the use of synthetic GH in the treatment of what is being called "somatotrophin deficiency syndrome" (SDS) in adults (somatotrophin is simply another term for GH). But what a conventional doctor calls a GH deficiency and what an antiaging physician calls one differ considerably. Conventional doctors will only offer GH to adults whose GH and IGF levels are low for their age. Antiaging doctors believe that GH and IGF levels that are normal for a young, healthy person should be maintained by all persons as they proceed into middle age to combat the unhealthy effects of a decreasing muscle mass and an increasing percentage of total body fat.

Because GH is a protein, it currently has to be injected; however, this is probably going to change soon. There are a number of research trials underway involving compounds that can be taken orally which can stimulate our pituitary glands to make and release more of our own GH. (It appears that the GH deficiency we suffer from as we age may not be because our pituitary becomes incapable of making and releasing GH, but simply because it is not stimulated *hard enough* to do so.) I suspect it will be only a short time before such compounds are available. Synthetic GH injections are also extremely expensive, and your health insurance will not pay for this. This is another good reason to wait for the oral GH-releasing compounds to be marketed.

Also, physical exercise is known to significantly increase pituitary release of GH in adults. So simply getting into a healthy, regular exercise program may defer any need you have for supplemental GH.

Melatonin

WHAT IT IS AND HOW IT WORKS

Melatonin is quite possibly the most amazing new substance available to the general public. An explosion of research on this molecule in the past decade has shown it to have a multitude of effects in animals and humans, even in plants and one-celled organisms. It may be one of the oldest molecules that exist in living creatures, having been found in every plant and animal searched to date. And whether it is found in a one-celled algae or a human being, the melatonin molecule seems to have the exact same structure, a phenomenon rarely seen in nature.

In humans, melatonin is produced in a tiny structure deep in the middle of the brain called the pineal gland, which releases the hormone into the blood primarily at night (some five to ten times as much of it is released during the night as during the day). Light turns out to be the critical factor; when daylight strikes our eyes, it conveys a message to the brain which blocks the production and release of melatonin. On the other hand, it takes sufficient amounts of exposure to light in the daytime to "prime" the pineal gland to produce melatonin at night. One study of women with premenstrual syndrome (PMS) demonstrated this by exposing them to two hours of particularly intense artificial light during the day; this group produced more melatonin at night and experienced improved mood. Other studies have shown that when people with seasonal affective disorder (SAD) are exposed to intense artificial light, their melatonin levels increase during the night, which corresponds to a decrease in their depression. To make the circle of light and melatonin complete, it turns out that exposure to artificial light *at night* can actually *decrease* melatonin production in humans. In fact, one study has shown that as little as five minutes of exposure to artificial light at night can inhibit melatonin production.

Thus, the message is clear: If we want to maximize our *natural* production of melatonin, we should get plenty of sunlight during the day; but on the other hand, it is important to keep your room as dark as possible at night to maximize production of melatonin.

Melatonin has been shown to promote restful sleep and the heightened energy that naturally follows from this. If you take healthy people and increase their blood melatonin levels in the middle of the day to the peak levels that occur in the middle of the night, this causes the onset of fatigue and sleepiness. This means that increased melatonin may be the natural physiological signal that initiates normal sleep onset in humans. And many studies suggest that high melatonin levels during the night not only promote deep sleep, but also aid in recovery; researchers see melatonin as a "repair" molecule that "fixes" much of the damage that accumulates in our bodies during the day.

Currently, when people have sleep problems, they are usually prescribed benzodiazepine drugs (such as Zanax, Halcion, and Valium) by their doctors, even though these drugs can produce a number of unwanted side effects, such as anxiety, depression, and memory loss. In addition, people often become resistant to these drugs, requiring ever increasing doses or a shift to another sleeping drug. As a treatment for insomnia, melatonin has no negative side effects, no toxicity (there has not yet been found a dose that can kill a rat), and it does not lose its effectiveness over time. It is currently believed that the elderly, who often have a number of sleep disorders, and may be taking many types of drugs, can benefit the most from melatonin in this regard.

Melatonin also appears to be very important in keeping our immune systems in top shape, being particularly effective in warding off the harmful effects that stress has on our immune system. Dr. George Maestron published a study in 1988 in which he took a group of mice and injected them with a sublethal dose of a virus that affects mice. Healthy mice can fight off the virus, but mice with a depleted immune system (such as occurs during chronic stress) have trouble combating the virus. After injecting the mice with the virus, Maestroni stressed them by confining them in a restraining device for a fixed amount of time. Some of the mice were then given melatonin. At the end of the study, 82 percent of the stressed-out mice who had *not* gotten melatonin died, while only 6 percent of the stressed-out mice who did receive melatonin died, almost a fourteenfold difference in survival.

As mentioned earlier, melatonin can neutralize hydroxyl free radicals, so it is believed also to help block the onset of cancer. Other evidence that demonstrates melatonin may prevent cancer is found in studies from Dr. Russ Reiter's laboratory at the University of Texas Health Science Center. Dr. Reiter has shown that if you take two groups of rats and inject both with the toxic substance safrole (which produces large amounts of free radicals) but inject one group with melatonin also, the amount of DNA damage present in liver cells twenty-four hours later is about 99 percent less in the rats which received melatonin. In addition, Dr. Reiter's group showed that if you expose human white blood cells to radiation, melatonin added to the cell cultures dramatically reduces the amount of damage to the cells' DNA.

Since the brain is particularly vulnerable to the hydroxyl free radical, and because melatonin readily enters into the brain after you ingest it, melatonin seems very attractive in minimizing long-term free radical damage to the brain, and the onset of neurodegenerative disease. This hormone is unique in that it is both water soluble and fat soluble. Therefore, it can work in the aqueous parts of the cell to halt free radicals as well as with the lipid parts, while other antioxidants are limited to one compartment of the cell or the other.

Melatonin may also help prevent heart disease. It maintains low blood-cholesterol levels in rats put on high cholesterol diets. New studies have shown that melatonin blocks cholesterol synthesis in human cells by as much as 38 percent. An ongoing study of melatonin as a contraceptive in humans has also suggested that it can help prevent heart disease. In Holland, fourteen hundred women have been taking very high doses of melatonin (about seventy-five milligrams) in order to block ovulation, and one of the interesting findings to come out of the study to date is that these women have experienced a 10 to 20 percent reduction in their blood-cholesterol levels. In addition, this same study has shown that women taking melatonin experience a decrease in blood pressure, a finding that has already been shown in animals. It goes without saying that lowering both cholesterol and blood pressure is important in ultimately avoiding heart disease.

Like all the hormones described in this chapter, melatonin gradually disappears from our blood and tissues as we age. In this case, it is because the pineal gland begins to shrivel up and calcify. Blood-melatonin levels stabilize after puberty, but then start their irreversible age-related decline in most of us at about the age of twenty-five. At age fifty, these levels begin to drop precipitously, so that by the time we are in our sixties, we only have about half as much of it circulating in our plasma as we did at twenty-five. This is not found so much in daytime blood levels of melatonin, but in the relative amounts of the late-night surges of it that we experience during youth.

DOSAGE

Melatonin should only be taken in the evening just before going to bed, the dosage based on its ability to help you easily get to sleep (or not interfere with your normal sleep, if you do not have sleeping problems), and to wake up feeling refreshed. For this purpose, doses range from .1 to 10 milligrams. Trial and error will tell you how much you can take without feeling sleepy the next day, the only known side effect of too large a dose. Likewise, experience will tell you how long before going to bed you should take it. Some people start to become drowsy within a half hour after taking melatonin, even in small amounts, while others need to take it up to two hours before retiring if it is going to have any sleep-inducing effect. I have found taking only .5 milligrams thirty minutes before going to bed puts me to sleep and lets me wake up refreshed. Any more than this gives me intense dreams, which tend to make me restless.

Melatonin also is very effective for jet lag. The dosage used by international flight crews is five milligrams just before bedtime, starting the first day of arrival at their destination, and continuing for five days after arriving. This causes a significant recovery in mood, energy, and alertness.

You can buy melatonin in pills, gelatin capsules, sublingual pills, or time-release capsules. The gelatin capsules and pills result in a large amount of melatonin being released into your bloodstream very quickly (less than an hour). Some of the melatonin will be metabolized when it passes through your liver after it is absorbed; but how much of it your liver metabolizes is extremely variable from person to person. You can purchase either synthetic or natural melatonin; I highly recommend the former. It is exactly the same structure as natural melatonin, but assuming the natural melatonin has been harvested from animal pineal glands, the synthetic hormone is less likely to be contaminated with any viruses or other animal pathogens.

It is probably best to buy the delayed-release melatonin capsules, as they more accurately mimic the delayed rise in melatonin from your pineal gland that occurs after you fall asleep. They can be found in many health food stores, or in sources listed at the back of this book.

Another way to increase your melatonin levels is to eat foods high in melatonin, or foods high in tryptophan, the melatonin-precursor molecule. Foods high in melatonin include oats, sweet corn, rice, tomatoes, bananas, and barley. Foods high in tryptophan include turkey, milk, soy nuts, cottage cheese, tofu, and almonds.

As one of the least expensive and easy-to-get hormone supplements, as well as one that is nontoxic in even high amounts, melatonin should be included in the Youthspan Extension Program of everyone over forty. The only exception are women who are pregnant, are breast-feeding, or are trying to become pregnant, as well as all men and women who have autoimmune disorders, kidney disease, or are taking the drug cortisone; no one in these groups should take melatonin without first consulting his or her physician. Interestingly, many antidepressant drugs increase the levels of melatonin in your blood. Yet a study published in the *British Journal of Psychiatry* in 1995 found that Prozac, one of the most popular antidepressants, actually decreases blood-melatonin levels, which may account for why many people who use it get insomnia. So it is recommended for Prozac users. But if you are taking any other antidepressant drugs, you probably should not take this hormone supplement.

People taking vitamin-B12 injections and those consuming lots of caffeine are also well advised to take melatonin supplements. Both B12 and caffeine seem to deplete melatonin levels. Also, special receptors called beta adrenergic receptors on the pineal gland must be activated for normal melatonin synthesis/release. So people chronically taking beta adrenergic receptor blocking drugs for hypertension or other cardiac problems (commonly known as beta blockers; for example, propranolol, labetalol, or timolol) make much less melatonin than normal, which may be one of the reasons these drugs cause insomnia in many who use them. These people should definitely take melatonin supplements.

CHAPTER ELEVEN

Muscle and Energy Tools II: Physical Exercise

*F*or the majority of Americans, it was not that long ago when physical activity was part of our daily routine, not something we had to make time for a couple of hours each week. We had to cut the firewood and drag it into the house. We often had to hunt game in order to eat. If we wanted to visit the neighbors, we walked or saddled up the horses for the long ride. We had to clear the land and plant the garden, and the kids had to walk to school, which was often many miles away. In those days, people got all the exercise (and then some) they wanted each day, and that kept their muscles firm, and their cardiovascular and respiratory systems functional well into old age. In addition, their bodies remained slim and firm, because the exercise not only allowed them to burn off calories every day, but also regulated their appetites and made their cells metabolize energy much more efficiently (which means not converting as much of their daily energy to fat).

True, the average lifespan was shorter back then because so many infectious diseases were fatal, particularly in children, and trauma therapy was almost nonexistent, but the ones who survived those things and lived to be elderly were in much better shape physically than most people over fifty nowadays.

How the times have changed.

In the last 100 years, technology ranging from the automobile to the reclining lounge chair have made our muscles an almost obsolete tissue. We have elevators and escalators so we don't have to bother with the tiresome stairs. We have all-terrain vehicles and snowmobiles so that when we want to get "back to Nature," we drive right up to Nature's doorstep. We have powerboats, so that when we want to go fishing or just get out on the lake, we don't have to deal with cumbersome oars or paddles. We have riding lawn mowers, automatic garage-door openers, remote channel changers so we don't even have to get out of the lounge chair to channel surf between games. And there are plenty of us who are still waiting for more technology to enable us to avoid those very few chores we still have to do without the help of a machine.

The first-ever Surgeon General's Report on Physical Activity and Health, released by the U.S. Centers for Disease Control and Prevention and the President's Council on Physical Fitness on the eve of the 1996 Centennial Olympic Games, shows that we are a nation of serious slackers. In this report, researchers followed more than 30,000 adult men and women for over eight years, tracking their fitness levels and monitoring risk factors for disease. It was found that sedentary individuals were one-and-a-half to two times more likely to die prematurely than those who were moderately fit. It was also concluded from this study that a sedentary lifestyle may even be a more serious health risk than high blood pressure, obesity, high cholesterol, or family history of disease—which I find to be a "circular" observation, since it is a lack of regular exercise itself that often leads to those very problems.

Exercise protects you against many of the things that shorten your Youthspan. Several clinical studies have shown that regular exercise provides dramatic benefits against the number one cause of age-related death, which is still cardiovascular disease. Exercise is also known to significantly decrease the incidence of colon cancer, and quite possibly breast cancer, and it improves the outlook in both Type-I and Type-II (noninsulin dependent) diabetes. Furthermore, it significantly improves mental health. In all, the scientific proof is so compelling, it is well worth taking a closer look at.

Exercise and Physical Strength and Mobility

A primary reason why older people become dependent is that their muscle mass, and therefore their strength, becomes drastically reduced by years of disuse. As we become weaker and weaker from decades of a sedentary life, we are unable to perform any physical tasks, from walking to the grocery store to enjoying healthy sex. Before long, we are no longer self-sufficient, and there is no greater indication of an aborted Youthspan than having to rely on others to assist you with your daily life. Obviously, physical exercise complements virtually every other aspect of this program. That old saw is true: Use it or lose it.

Not only does exercise reduce fat and increase muscle mass and endurance on its own, but it also causes us to release bursts of GH from our pituitary gland into our blood. Therefore, the benefits of exercise on our muscle mass alone (and therefore our appearance as well as our strength) are twofold; a direct strengthening of our muscles and joints, and a release of GH from our pituitary glands which will further promote muscle growth and function, and decrease body fat.

And it is never too late to start. It has been clearly shown in many studies that if we engage in a regimen of resistance-exercise training when we are older, we can still experience a significant increase in muscle strength. This is important not only from a standpoint of remaining independent, but also for overall health, as age-related muscle atrophy from muscle disuse is a big contributor to the high incidence of injurious falls in old age.

Recently, studies from Tufts University have shown that men and women over age fifty-six who participated in a strength-building exercise program, working out in three thirty-minute sessions per week for twelve weeks, on average increased their strength by 24 percent and decreased their body fat by 3 percent. Furthermore, this exercise increased their basal metabolism—how fast and efficiently they burn calories while at rest. One result is that participants are able to consume an extra 300 calories a day without gaining weight.

Exercise and the Cardiovascular System

The cardiovascular system encompasses your heart, as well as the blood vessels that your heart pumps blood through. Damage to either will result in an inability to supply tissues with nutrients and oxygen, and prevent waste products from being removed from the tissues which ultimately will damage or kill them.

Physical exercise, fortunately, can prevent several common causes of cardiovascular disease. In fact, the only factor in cardiovascular disease it can't help is the disease's most preventable cause: smoking.

Hypertension (High Blood Pressure)

Having your blood pressure checked by your physician annually is an extremely important part of having a long Youthspan, because you can find out if you need to take steps to control it, before it takes steps that will ultimately control you. Fortunately, exercise may alleviate hypertension in a number of ways, such as by decreasing the activity of the sympathetic nervous system, or by increasing the release of certain blood-pressure–lowering peptide proteins from the heart and blood vessels. In addition, some of the reasons that exercise decreases blood pressure may be secondary to the fact that exercise reduces stress (see below), which is well known to elevate blood pressure. Another very good reason to control blood pressure is that chronically high blood pressure can result in the rupture of small capillaries in the brain, and produce a form of dementia.

Serum Lipids

It is well known that high blood levels of lipids such as apolipoproteins (especially apolipoproteins A and B), cholesterol (particularly LDL), and special fats known as "triglycerides" promote atherosclerosis. This occurs when certain types of lipids and other substances accumulate in the cells which line our arteries. When these cellular deposits start to "bulge out" into the space within the artery, they

148

squeeze off blood moving through the artery, and deprive whatever tissue is downstream of that artery of its normal blood supply.

Very often the arteries that get clogged during atherosclerosis are the coronary arteries, which supply the heart muscle with blood. When this happens, the heart muscle becomes slowly deprived of blood, and if it is deprived long enough, heart cells begin to die. At some point you would begin to feel chest pain, and you might even have a heart attack. This process of deprivation is called "ischemic heart disease" (ischemia is a medical term describing inadequate arterial blood flow to any tissue), and it kills us by the thousands each year. But the important thing to remember here is that even if you don't have a fatal heart attack, any heart tissue that was killed due to a prolonged lack of blood supply is now gone for good. So even if you start making corrections to alter your cholesterol levels in a favorable direction at this point, you may have already lost some of your functional heart tissue permanently. Which is why you need to do something about your blood cholesterol and lipoprotein profile *now*.

Fortunately, aerobic exercise (exercise that causes you to increase your heart and respiratory rates for a prolonged period of time) can increase HDL (good cholesterol) and decrease LDL as well as triglycerides.

Exercise and Diabetes

There are two major types of diabetes: Type II (or 'adult onset') and Type I. Type-II diabetes is a condition where the cell receptors that normally respond to insulin don't work well anymore, resulting in chronically high levels of both blood glucose and insulin: the high blood-glucose level stimulates the pancreas to crank out more insulin, which can't move the glucose from the blood to the cells, so even more insulin is produced. This vicious cycle is extremely unhealthy, particularly for the cardiovascular system. In Type-I diabetes, the pancreas can't make insulin at all (probably due to an autoimmune disorder that destroys the insulin-producing cells in the pancreas), also often resulting in cardiovascular disease due to chronically high glucose levels. Type-I diabetics usually have to take insulin injections for their entire lives to control their blood glucose.

In addition to coping with cardiovascular disease, persons with Type-I or Type-II diabetes suffer from a variety of problems as they go through life, including peripheral neuropathies (painful sensations in their limbs), decreased blood flow to the extremities (often resulting in amputations), cataracts, loss of vision, and complete kidney failure. Most of these problems are related to the fact that chronically high levels of blood glucose over decades wreak havoc with all sorts of cells. The message is clear: Although we need glucose as a source of energy, maintaining high blood levels of it for long periods of time can kill us early in life.

Fortunately, exercise can help us greatly in our endeavor to maintain healthy levels of blood glucose. Acute (intense) exercise tends to increase the effectiveness of insulin, and therefore can reduce the levels of blood glucose in both Type-I and Type-II diabetics. But even light exercise produces a significant improvement in glucose levels.

Recent studies show it is never too late for diabetics to benefit from exercise. One study of postmenopausal women (aged fifty to sixty-five years) with Type II diabetes showed that using exercise machines just three times a week for four months significantly increased their physical strength, as well as the effectiveness of their insulin, thereby reducing the high levels of insulin and glucose present in many of these women. The authors concluded that not only does exercise appear to be very helpful in lessening problems associated with Type-II diabetes in persons that have it, but *it may also help prevent Type-II diabetes from occurring in the first place.* A similar finding was also recorded recently in older men.

Exercise for Stress and Depression

Anyone who has ever exercised regularly knows that getting a good physical workout decreases levels of anxiety. It does so at least partly by promoting the release of a substance called "beta endorphin," as well as other opioids into our brain and blood; these are Nature's natural painkillers and relaxers.

Depression is a more serious problem than stress. Depression may be bipolar (meaning you are depressed at times and manic at others), unipolar (depressed all the time), or situational (depressed lots of the time, but not always). Depression is the most commonly diagnosed mental disorder in the United States, and is twice as prevalent in women as it is in men. Diagnostic criteria include poor appetite, significant weight loss (or excessive eating with weight gain), insomnia (or hypersomnia), hyperactivity (or listlessness), feelings of worthlessness and inappropriate guilt, and recurring thoughts of death and suicide.

Depression is believed to be caused by a reduction in the release of the neurotransmitters serotonin and norepinephrine in the brain; antidepressant drugs work by increasing their levels. Happily, like stress, depression responds well to regular aerobic exercise. We don't know exactly how exercise alleviates the symptoms of depression, but it may be that somehow it stimulates the release of those key neurotransmitters. What we do know, however, is that exercise increases alpha-wave activity, the brain waves most associated with relaxed wakefulness.

Dr. Kathleen Moore, a health psychologist at Duke University Medical Center, reported recently that preliminary results from an ongoing major study on depression showed that short—as little as eight minutes at a time—but strenuous workouts can dramatically reduce symptoms of depression. The participants, all of whom were suffering with diagnosed depression, reported an overall 82 percent reduction in feelings of depression, fatigue, anger, and confusion after the exercise. Dr. Moore stated that exercise may be an adjunct therapy for treating depression, and that "this is particularly important for older adults who may want to limit the number of medications they take to control a multitude of medical problems."

Exercise and Cancer

Animal studies and human epidemiolgical studies have long suggested that there is an inverse relationship between regular exercise and the incidence of cancer. Colon cancer in particular, still the second most common and fatal type of cancer among adults, has been positively correlated with a history of low physical exercise.

So has breast cancer, a leading cause of mortality in women. The first proof that women who exercise regularly may decrease breast cancer came in 1985, when it was noted that the incidence

151

of this cancer was lower in women who had been athletes in college. Further epidemiological studies that followed also demonstrated a lower risk of other types of cancer in women who had been athletic in college. A 1997 study regarding exercise and breast cancer that was reported in the *Journal of the American Medical Association* derived its data from over 25,000 women in Norway (aged twenty to fifty-four years), who were followed for nearly fourteen years during the mid- to late 1970s. The study found that those women who regularly engaged in physical exercise (especially if it was for four hours a week or more) had a significantly smaller likelihood of developing breast cancer, particularly if they were premenopausal.

It is still not known exactly how exercise prevents cancer from developing because exercise affects so many physiological systems. However, one suggestion has been that exercise may increase the immune system's ability to detect cancers early and kill cancer cells before they get a chance to grow. Also, regular, vigorous exercise can decrease the regularity of menstrual cycles, and therefore may result in less exposure to high circulating levels of estrogen in regularly exercising women (although estrogen does not seem to cause cancer directly, it can enhance the growth of some types of cancer if they should arise in the body).

Exercise and Immunity

The adaptive immune system can essentially be divided into two aspects: cell mediated and humoral. The cell-mediated aspect is composed of specific cells that coordinate attacks on foreign invaders: the T lymphocytes, leukocytes, "natural killer" (NK) cells, etc.; the humoral part is composed of the antibodies, which are special proteins made by a type of lymphocyte called "B cells." Antibodies are often used to immediately seek out and "tag" foreign substances, so the T cells and other cells can later find them more easily and kill them.

There is no question that many parameters of the adaptive immune system are changed after an acute bout of exercise. However, different results are found depending on whether you are looking at humoral or cell-mediated responses, at younger or older people, and whether or not the people are generally physically fit. In relatively young people who are generally sedentary, riding an exercise bicycle to exhaustion can increase a number of important lymphocytes and leukocytes circulating in the blood. And when researchers look at the NK cells, they often see an increase in their number and activity after exercise. For example, a 1989 study found that an acute bout of exercise increased NK activity in a group of both young and older women. In addition, a study involving four months of aerobic training with elderly women (average age, seventy-two years) showed elevated resting values of NK cell activity that were 33 percent higher than the nonexercising control group.

The effects of long-term exercise training on humoral immunity have yielded mixed results. Although it has been shown that antibody levels do not change dramatically in marathon runners after a race, moderate brisk walking does increase the levels of certain antibodies. So, although several studies have shown that people who are not top-flight athletes undergo beneficial immune changes after exercising, other studies have not shown any significant changes in humoral or cell-mediated immunity after chronic or acute exercise.

Exercise and Sleep

Sleep complaints represent one of the most common difficulties experienced by older adults. Even though they account for only about 15 percent of the current adult population in the United States, older Americans received 35 to 40 percent of the prescriptions for sedative/hypnotic drugs, mostly on a long-term basis. However, these drugs can be particularly troublesome for older people, as they can readily cause confusion, falls, extended drowsiness, and potentially harmful interactions with other drugs. Happily, recent studies show that regular exercise, consisting merely of brisk walking and low-impact aerobics three or four times a week, produces significant improvements in the ability to sleep well.

Physical Exercise and Your Healthy Brain

There is another very exciting aspect of physical exercise that has come to light lately: exercise affects the health of our brains. Epidemiological studies show that physically fit men and women perform better on cognitive tests than their sedentary peers, increasingly so as they age.

Nonetheless, it has not yet been proven that physical exercise protects the brain from disease, although some studies have shown that the declines in cerebral blood flow that occur with aging are prevented in individuals who remain physically active into their later years. Another promising mechanism, "neurotrophic factors," has been discovered recently in animals that may explain how physical exercise mitigates against age-related brain damage. These compounds nourish the mammalian brain, provide it with long-term maintenance, and help neurons form new and more functional synapses with other neurons. It is now known that physical exercise significantly increases the synthesis of several of these nerve-growth factors in cognitive-functioning areas in mammalian brains. When you consider that these neurotrophic factors are critical for normal cognitive functioning, and that many of them decline with age, physical exercise appears to be a good bet for maintaining brain health.

Physical Exercise Methods

When it comes to physical exercise programs, there are more books and videos and health club routines out there than you can throw a barbell at. As far as I can tell, most of them are quite good, and generally I would be hard pressed to recommend one over another. But what I can do is help you make an educated choice about what program to choose—take the program that you are most likely to regularly stick to—and I can provide you with a few basic principles of physical exercise.

As always, prior to beginning an exercise program you should get a complete physical examination, including an exercise treadmill test with electrocardiogram monitoring.

TYPES OF EXERCISE

There are essentially two types of exercise that everyone who is physically able should be performing: aerobic and anaerobic (also called resistance exercise or weight training). Essentially, aerobic exercise gives your heart and lungs a workout, increasing your pulse rate and your consumption of oxygen, while anaerobic exercise is aimed at increasing muscular strength and endurance. Most of the health benefits discussed above accrue from aerobic exercise, although resistance training, when done properly, has been shown to increase plasma-growth-hormone levels more than aerobic exercise does. But in general the value of anaerobic exercise should not be underestimated: maintaining muscle strength prevents many of the mobility problems associated with old age. Another benefit of resistance training is that muscle tissue burns calories more effectively than fat (adipose) tissue, so maintaining more muscle mass lets our bodies dispose of calories more efficiently, preventing us from becoming overweight. And, of course, anaerobic exercise improves our physical appearance which, in itself, can go a long way to boosting our mood.

HOW TO START

Although there are several aerobic exercises that can be done quite effectively on one's own (such as walking or jogging), far and away your best bet for making significant gains is to join a regular health club. These can be found in almost all areas of the country and are generally quite affordable. Most health clubs have trainers who will design a specific aerobic and anaerobic exercise program for you, and will show you how to properly use the exercise equipment. (I definitely recommend against resistance training at home because of the possibility of injury.) Health clubs also provide psychological support, showing you that you can really do what you set out to do. And the cost of joining can be a prime motivator in keeping you going on a regular basis.

BASICS OF AEROBIC EXERCISING

Aerobic exercising consists of a warm-up phase, a conditioning phase (when you actually do most of the exercising), and a cool-down phase. Exercising is stressful to our muscles, hence the warm-up phase where we stretch our muscles and get blood flowing into them to avoid tissue injury. The cool-down phase helps the muscles return to their resting level of activity; walking and/or light stretching after the conditioning phase will help prevent postexercise muscle cramping.

The conditioning phase is further subcategorized for its intensity, duration, and frequency. Intensity is the level of effort you put into your workout, duration is the amount of time a single workout lasts, and frequency is how often you exercise. The currently recommended training frequency for maximal benefits from aerobic exercising is three to five times per week, with a duration of more than twenty continuous minutes. That is why exercises like golfing and bowling are not particularly good aerobic exercises: we never go twenty minutes without stopping. And that's why exercises like taking a long walk, jogging, swimming, and dancing are much more aerobically healthy.

THE TARGET HEART RATE

The most important factor in the conditioning phase of an aerobic-exercise program is the intensity of the exercise you do. To get maximum benefits for your long-term health, you need to increase your heart rate from its resting level to 50 to 80 percent of what is known as your functional capacity, or your "maximum heart rate" (MHR), for twenty minutes or more; this is your Target Heart Rate. You will know what your MHR is if you have had an exercise treadmill test done; if not, you can roughly estimate your MHR by subtracting your age from 220.

For many of you, it may be too cumbersome to try to take your pulse during a workout, so I suggest you purchase a *heart-rate monitor,* a simple device that measures your heart rate in a digital readout. These monitors can be purchased at almost any exercise or fitness stores, including places that sell bicycles. They can also be ordered from fitness magazines, like *Runner's World.*

For those of you who are already thinking of excuses for not exercising, like the time-honored "I never have the time," let me just say that walking even short distances is an excellent aerobic workout.

Start out by walking three times a week. Bring your heart monitor, or a watch with a second hand, to calculate how fast you have to walk and for how long to get your heart rate up into the lower part of your target heart range; it should only take a few days of experimenting to figure this out. Then you will be ready to stay in that range for at least twenty minutes. After a few weeks, increase both your duration and your intensity so you can bring your heart rate further up into your target range. Allow five to ten minutes to cool down after your walk.

Note: Be sure to wear comfortable clothing and to stretch before starting. In summer, walk early in the morning or late in the evening to avoid excess heat production.

This or any aerobic-exercise program can be summarized as progressive, with gradual increases in intensity and duration, and a goal of reaching an intensity of 70 percent of the target heart rate for thirty to forty-five minutes, three to four times a week. Your body will tell you if you are doing too much exercise; if aches and pains in your joints become a problem, cut back and, of course, if you experience any chest pains, see your physician immediately.

BASICS OF ANAEROBIC EXERCISING

Just like an aerobic-exercise program, an anaerobic program should *weights.* include a warm-up period before starting and a cool-down period after finishing. Resistance training to increase strength focuses on essentially four components: 1) the number of bouts (sets); 2) the number of repetitions done per bout; 3) the quantity of weight lifted; and 4) the rest period between bouts.

The number of repetitions you do makes a big difference in whether you maximize your muscle strength or your muscle endurance. For example, if you are lifting a weight so heavy that you can only do six or fewer repetitions, this exercise is more effective for development of muscular strength; if the amount of weight you are lifting is low enough to allow you to do twenty or more repetitions, this is more effective in developing muscle endurance. And amount of weight that allows for between eight and fifteen repetitions is effective for the development of both and is unlikely to result in muscle soreness or injury. *How*

After learning proper lifting technique, your initial selection of weight should be based on your being able to perform *eight repetitions* of the exercise, with at least two of them requiring a concerted effort. The number of sets used in a workout is generally three, and the length of time between sets is usually one to three minutes. Thus, if the goal is to increase muscular strength, longer rest periods (at least three minutes) are used between sets. If the goal is to increase muscle endurance, rest periods of one minute or less are used between sets.

In addition to the rest allowed between sets, it is important to consider the order of the exercises. Following an arm exercise with a leg exercise is useful to some people who are just starting, as it gives the arm muscles some recovery time while the legs are being exercised. Many people, myself induced, like to do all arm and upper body exercises on one day, and all leg and lower body exercises on other days.

Resistance-training sessions are usually conducted three times per week, with at least one day between each workout. Since there are tremendous benefits to both resistance- and aerobic-exercise training, the ultimate goal is to work out six days a week, with resistance and aerobic exercises on alternate days. It really can make a huge difference in your health if you can just make the time to do it, and do it properly.

Note: Don't think for a minute that you are ever too old to start resistance exercises. In the Elder Hostel Program at my university, I have watched many older people start off in a resistance program with very low muscle strength, only to see it increase dramatically by the end of the summer. The scientific literature is filled with studies showing significant strength improvement in elderly people who start properly run resistance-exercise programs.

CHAPTER TWELVE

Muscle and Energy Tools III: Diet

Obesity Dramatically Decreases Youthspan and Lifespan

*E*ating too many calories, especially if many of those calories come from foods high in saturated fat, results in a serious detour from a long Youthspan because it almost always leads to obesity, the second most preventable cause of death in this country, right behind smoking. A diagnosis of obesity is determined by phy- calculate sicians by calculating your "body mass index" (BMI, your weight in kilograms divided by the square of your height in meters). A BMI of 27.8 kg/M^2 is defined as overweight in adult men, and a BMI of 27.3 kg/M^2 is overweight in adult women. This does not apply to people with an exceptionally high muscle mass, such as weight lifters and some football players. A BMI of 30 kg/M^2 or greater is defined as obesity in both men and women.

Currently, more than one-third of all adult Americans are obese. Regardless of how obese people feel about their physical appearance, their obesity is a major risk factor for high blood pressure, heart dis- ease, diabetes, gallbladder disease, and breast, colon, and other can- cers, and it contributes to more than 300,000 deaths annually in the United States. Obesity also aggravates existing problems such as arthri- tis. Everyone knows that the health care industry is in financial trouble, but not everyone realizes that billions and billions of dollars are spent each year to take care of people with health problems caused by obesity.

The food industry continues to make unhealthy living very easy. Fast-food restaurants and doughnut shops have sprouted up all across the country in the last three decades, contributing mightily to our waistline expansion and Youthspan contraction. Another reason we are getting fatter is that Americans are currently on a "fat-free" frenzy. When we see "fat-free" on a box of cookies, we assume that means calorie-free, which of course it doesn't. Calories from carbohydrates and proteins can also be converted to fat by our bodies, if you eat enough of them.

Obesity is a serious enough problem in adults who develop it later in life, but the development of obesity in our children is particularly insidious. Obesity is occurring in our kids faster than ever; studies show that the rate of obesity occurring in children six to eleven years old has increased more than 50 percent over the last fifteen years. The chance that a child will become obese as an adult is 80 percent if both parents are obese, 40 percent if one parent is obese, and 7 percent if neither parent is obese. Most people tend to think that this is completely due to genetics, and that they can do nothing about it, but that is just not true. Genetics does play a role in obesity, but quite often obesity is a product of one's environment. For example, some scientists believe that one reason for the dramatic rise in childhood obesity is a general increase in sedentary activity among children (watching television), combined with an increasingly greater calorie and fat intake (eating potato chips while watching television). In addition, if a child's parents are obese, chances are these parents don't exercise, and regularly serve high-fat meals with little or not fruits and vegetables. Little Junior is just role modeling.

A Little Off Goes a Long Way

If you are struggling with a weight problem, you should know that even a moderate decrease in your weight results in a significant increase in your health. This was clearly shown in the Nurses Health Study, in which more than 115,000 nurses were followed for more than sixteen years. In this study, the risk of death was 60 to 70 percent higher among those nurses who had a BMI between 29 and 32, compared to those with a BMI between 25 and 27. What this translates into is 1,260 excess lives lost per million women per year as a consequence of an average weight difference of only thirteen kilograms (about twenty-eight pounds). This is a very good reason to start trying to lose at least some weight right now and to learn how to keep it off. As anyone who has ever dieted knows, dieting does not work, and more than 95 percent of the people who go on a rapid-weight-loss diet regain the lost weight in less than two years. Depriving yourself of food simply tells your body you are starving, and it will then do everything it can to fight this weight loss, including metabolizing what calories you do eat less rapidly, decreasing your body temperature, increasing your appetite, and programming your tissues to store fat at an increased rate once you start eating regularly again (which almost every dieter eventually does). In addition, some studies have shown that dieting in this way is actually harmful to your health.

True weight control requires a lifestyle change, which means losing weight slowly over time (so your body does not think you are starving), regular exercise (which is very important in burning and storing calories in a beneficial way and in controlling appetite), and choosing the right combination of foods for your body.

There are always going to be overweight people who will try to lose pounds this way but will fail, either because of their lack of willpower or an abnormal physiology. For those individuals, the possibility of using medications to help lose weight should be discussed with their doctor. Some of these drugs may be harmful to certain people, and many readers may be aware of the serious heart and lung side effects that have occurred in some users of "fen-phen," a combination of the prescription appetite-suppressing drugs fenfluramine and phentermine, which resulted in the removal of fenfluramine from the United States market by FDA in 1997.

However, there are dugs other than fenfluramine which can be tried in weight management. Be sure to have your doctor clearly explain the risks of any drugs she might prescribe, weighed against the significant health benefits of shedding excessive pounds.

Is How Much You Eat Killing You?

Even if you are not clinically obese, eating far more calories each day than your body actually needs to keep functioning can significantly shorten both your lifespan and your Youthspan. A study done over sixty years ago demonstrated that if you feed two groups of animals well-balanced diets, but restrict the total calories that one group consumes, they will live longer and with far fewer health problems than the animals that are allowed to eat all the calories they wanted. And this occurs even if the animals eating all those extra calories do not become obese. I am not talking about buying a few extra days of life here; many of these studies found that the animals with a limited calorie intake consistently live up to one-third or more longer than their well-fed counterparts. Furthermore, I am not talking about starvation diets—the animals on restricted caloric intake do not lose weight. The idea is to supply them with only enough calories to run their metabolic machinery and support all the energy-using life-functions going on in their bodies, along with the energy needed to support their daily physical activity.

If this relationship between decreased total caloric intake and in-creased lifespan/Youthspan applies to humans (and there is evidence that it does), a calorie-restricted diet represents one way we can live young much longer. The "Gompertz Mortality Rate Model," a mathe-matical model used to predict the rate at which we age and die, indi-cates that if the rate of mortality-reduction achieved in animals through caloric restriction were applied to humans, *the median human life expectancy would approach 120 years!* This could add up to some serious quality time spent with your great-grandchildren.

And there is more good news. These animals don't just live longer, they live *young* longer. Caloric restriction has been clearly shown to dramatically retard the onset of kidney disease, heart disease, cancers such as lymphoma and leukemia, and autoimmune disease in many different strains of rats and mice. In addition, animals that have re-stricted caloric intake over a large part of their lives show far fewer symptoms of memory disorders than animals that eat unrestricted calories.

Now evidence is starting to accumulate that caloric restriction plays a major role in extending the Youthspan of humans. A small group of people involved in a project called Biosphere II lived in a closed ecosystem where they consumed an average energy intake of just over 1,700 calories per day from the food they grew in the biosphere. Over the first six months of the project, they reported a significant fall in body weight, blood pressure, triglycerides, total cholesterol, and fasting blood glucose, all changes reported in calorie-restricted rodents who experienced an increased Youthspan.

There are some populations that just normally eat fewer calories than most others. For example, on the Japanese island of Okinawa, detailed studies have shown that dietary energy intake for adults is about 20 percent less than the average for the rest of Japan. In addition, school children there consume only about 62 percent of the dietary energy intake recommended in Japan. And guess what? The incidence of centenarians on Okinawa is twenty to forty times that of other Japanese islands. Also, death rates from cerebral vascular disease, malignancy, and heart disease are only 59 percent, 69 percent, and 59 percent, respectively, of the average for the rest of Japan.

How Caloric Intake Is Related to Increased Lifespan and Youthspan

Most scientists believe that it comes down to free radicals again, that if you reduce the total number of calories that you ingest daily over many years, you will reduce the number of dangerous oxygen free radicals produced in your cell's mitochondria each day over many years. Thus, lowered production of oxygen free radicals = less cellular damage = increased Youthspan and lifespan. Indeed, animal studies show that eating calorie-restricted diets specifically decreases oxygen-free-radical damage to cell membranes as well as to cellular DNA. Other theories revolving around free radicals may also explain why caloric restriction increases the lifespan and Youthspan of animals. For example, it has been shown that in some tissues of aging animals, the effectiveness and/or quantity of the important cellular antioxidant enzymes returns to youthful levels if the animals are put on calorie-restricted diets.

How to Determine Your Minimal Daily Calorie Requirement

What is the minimal amount of energy in the form of calories your body actually needs daily in order for you to stay alive and functional? Knowing something about what factors contribute to how many total calories you require each day helps you understand how to modify your daily caloric intake to come close to this number, and scientists have devised ways to calculate this minimum number.

One of the major energy requiring processes in our bodies is referred to as the *basal metabolic rate,* or BMR. The BMR is the energy we burn while seated or lying at rest in a comfortable environment. We may not think we are burning calories if we are at rest, but we have to in order to provide energy for all the biological functions our bodies are performing constantly. These normal body functions include such things as breathing, forming waste products, circulating blood, conducting nerve impulses, and secreting hormones, and together they account for 60 to 75 percent of our daily energy needs.

VARIATIONS IN THE BMR

So why do some of us burn more calories at rest than others? Everyone has a friend who eats like a horse, never exercises, but never gains a pound. Or, on the other hand, we all know people who eat very small quantities of food, yet constantly put on weight. Assuming that these people all absorb the food they eat at approximately the same rates and efficiency from their digestive tract, the reason for this phenomenon must be that some people simply burn up calories more efficiently when they are resting, instead of storing the extra calories from their food as fat.

Some of the factors that are known to influence the BMR in adults are body size, age, gender, thyroid hormone status, sympathetic nervous system activity, pregnancy, fever, and medical disorders such as cancer and burns. Most significant is that scientists have found that the amount of "lean body mass" present in the body is directly related to the BMR. Since lean body mass is essentially muscle, this is why maintaining a high lean body mass (through exercising) as you age helps you to maintain a more ideal body weight; muscle cells simply burn energy faster and more efficiently than do fat cells.

In addition to BMR calories, we need calories to provide energy for our muscles when we move around or exercise. Since we are all individuals with different levels of daily activity, those calories needed for activity (called the thermic effect of exercise, or TEE) must be calculated on an individualized basis.

CALCULATION OF THE BMR

Nutritional scientists have developed an equation, the *Harris-Benedict Equation,* which can be used to accurately estimate the BMR. This is used by physicians, clinical nutritionists, and registered dietitians to estimate the energy needs (measured in calories) of persons requiring calorie-controlled diets (such as weight loss/gain diets, or intravenous/tube feedings). It works as follows:

Calculated BMR for Men

$$66 + (13.7 \times \text{weight in kilograms}) + (5 \times \text{height in centimeters}) - (6.8 \times \text{age in years})$$

Calculated BMR for Women

$$655 + (9.6 \times \text{weight in kilograms}) + (1.8 \times \text{height in centimeters}) - (\times 4.7 \times \text{age in years})$$

You can convert your weight from pounds to kilograms simply by dividing your weight in pounds by 2.2. To convert your height in inches to height in centimeters, simply multiply your height in inches times 2.54.

ESTIMATION OF THE TEE

Now that we have calculated our BMR, we must estimate the number of calories we require each day for our physical activity, our TEE. In most persons, the TEE represents the second largest component of energy output (unless you are competing in a triathlon every day) and usually accounts for 15 to 30 percent of total energy expenditure in persons who are moderately active. Because the energy needed to perform different types of activities can vary greatly, TEE usually differs considerably among individuals, and also within the same person from day to day.

Your TEE can be easily altered by simply changing your activity level. If you start exercising more, you increase your TEE, burn more calories, and promote control of body weight (since most of us eat too many calories daily, not too few). To estimate what your TEE is, a TEE "activity factor" is determined, according to which of the five daily activity patterns below best categorizes your daily activity:

- sedentary
- very light
- light
- moderate
- heavy

Sedentary: Your activity factor for calculating TEE is 20 percent of your BMR. This factor should be used if you spend most of your day sitting with minimal movement. This would include sitting or reclining while watching television, listening to music, or reading or resting while seated or reclining, and sleeping.

Very Light: Your activity factor is 30 percent of your BMR. This factor should be used if you spend most of your day doing seated or standing activities that require fairly low activity physical movements, and if you also do not participate in any higher energy activities such as exercising, recreational activities, or household work.

As a point of reference, this activity level means that out of the 24 hours in a day you spend about 10 hours per day at rest, and about 14 hours per day doing very light activities. Very light activities include driving, typing, writing, word processing, computer programming, laboratory work, seated assembly line work, sewing, painting, ironing, cooking, personal care, and rocking in a chair. Recreational activities in this category include playing cards, billiards, or a musical instrument.

Light: Your activity factor is 60 percent of your BMR if you're a man, and 50 percent of your BMR if you're a women. This level (and the "moderate" level which follows it) is a typical activity pattern for many persons living in the U.S. This activity factor should be used if you spend most of your day doing activities that require you to be somewhat mobile, but also use your upper body. Light activities include household chores such as washing clothes, sweeping floors, washing the car, light landscaping, and making beds, work such auto repair or garage work, house painting, store clerk, bagger, or stocker, electrical trades, carpentry, restaurant work, standing assembly line work, or child care.

Recreational activities include walking at 2 to 3 mph (equals 20 to 30 minutes per mile) on a level surface, bicycling at 5 to 6 mph on a level surface, bowling, golfing (with cart), sailing, easy canoeing, and playing table tennis or softball.

Moderate: Your activity factor is 70 percent of your BMR if you are a man, and 60 percent of your BMR if you are a woman. As mentioned above, this is also a typical activity pattern for persons living in the U.S. This factor should be used if you spend most of your day at an occupation that requires significant walking and/or physical labor. These moderate activities include occupations such as construction work (this can vary from moderate to heavy depending on specific duties), landscaping (such as light digging, pulling weeds, or pushing a nonself-propelled mower), walking while carrying a load on a level surface such as a mailman or longshoreman, standing assembly line work involving lifting and walking (this can vary according to specific work type), and farming.

Recreational activities include walking at 3 to 4 mph or on hills/stairs, bicycling at 8 to 9 mph or on hills, moderate-intensity aerobics, dancing, ballet, doubles tennis, golfing (no cart), hard canoeing or kayaking, water skiing, roller-blading, or playing volleyball.

Heavy: Your activity factor is 110 percent of your BMR if you are a man, and 90 percent of your BMR if you are a woman. This factor should be used if you spend most of your day at an occupation that requires significant walking or hard physical labor. These heavy activities can include occupations such as construction work and outdoor work such as heavy manual digging, chopping wood/felling trees, shoveling snow, and walking while carrying a load up hills. Recreational activities can include jogging/running at 5 mph (or greater) and on hills/stairs, bicycling at 11 to 12 mph and on hills, heavy-intensity aerobics, vigorous swimming, rock climbing or vigorous hiking over rocks/hills, cross-country or downhill skiing, playing singles tennis, racquetball, basketball, soccer, or ice hockey.

Once you have calculated your BMR and determined which activity pattern best matches your usual level of activity, you can calculate the number of calories you need each day to meet your minimal daily energy requirements.

For example

Suppose you are a forty-two-year-old male who is six feet tall (sixty inches) and weighs 190 pounds. To calculate your BMR, you would first convert your height to centimeters and your weight to kilograms. In this case, you would be 152 centimeters tall and weigh 86 kilograms. Plugging these values into the Harris-Benedict equation for males (above) would tell you that you need to consume approximately 1,718 calories each day even if you did no physical activity at all.

Now let us assume this same man is a construction worker and therefore has an activity level that is considered moderate. By looking at the above information on TEE activity factors, we would estimate this individual's TEE to be approximately 70 percent of his BMR, which is 1,202 calories. Therefore, this man would require a total of approximately 2,920 calories each day to simply run his daily biochemical reactions, and to support his daily level of physical activity. In other words, any calories he consumes above and beyond 2,920 calories each day are "excess" calories for him, which can be used to generate excess oxygen free radicals, or could potentially be stored as fat.

Please be aware that as of fall of 1997, there is a site on the Internet where you can download software for personal computers which can do the above calculations for you, as well as provide other very useful health information, such as the nutrient composition of various foods, metric conversions, and how to calculate body mass index. Check out this website at http://www.lisp.com.au/~david_t/index.htm.

THE REAL WORLD

I want to be realistic with the reader about calculating a minimal daily caloric requirement, and trying to eat only that number of calories each day. Although it certainly appears that restricting excess caloric intake beyond what is minimally needed by your body is a potentially powerful tool in the battle to increase our Youthspan, it certainly is not easy. We humans enjoy our food, and lots of it. Therefore, look at your estimated minimal daily caloric requirement as a guideline, and attempt to eat as close to this number of total calories each day as is possible for you. For some people, shooting for this minimal intake of calories every other day, or every other week, is an acceptable goal. Few if any people will be able to restrict their total daily caloric intake to the calculated minimal amount, so you have to try it and see how well you do personally. Do not attempt to restrict your daily caloric intake to the point where you get frustrated, and give up on it completely.

Practicing daily total caloric restriction should only be done by adults and never by people who are not yet fully grown (individuals under the age of around 22). In addition, total caloric restriction should never be used by people who have pre-existing health problems, especially metabolic disorders like diabetes. And if you have ever experienced an eating disorder such as anorexia or bulimia, you should not practice daily total caloric restriction.

Finally, now that you know how to estimate the minimal number of calories that your body requires each day, you have to consider the composition of those calories. In other words, if you determined your minimal daily energy requirement was 2,000 calories, you certainly would not want 75 percent of those calories coming from fat. So let's now consider what would be an optimal nutrient profile to get from our total daily caloric intake.

The nutrients that you consume to get your daily calories ultimately come from three sources: proteins, fats, and carbohydrates (CHO). Proteins are made up of compounds called amino acids; when we eat proteins, these amino acids are released in our small intestine and are then absorbed into the bloodstream from which our own cells take them up and use them to assemble our own proteins inside the cell. Fats in our diet supply us with the essential fatty acids and lipids we need to maintain healthy cell membranes in all our cells, and to manufacture certain types of hormones. And the carbohydrates in our diet are used as the predominant source of glucose, which is the main blood sugar that cells use to make energy in the form of ATP. Although CHOs are primarily used in the body as an energy source, proteins and fats can also supply the body with energy.

The amount of calories provided by the carbohydrates, protein, and fat we eat varies. For example, one gram of CHO contains approximately four calories, as does one gram of protein. But one gram of fat provides about nine calories, more than twice as many calories as a gram of CHO or protein. Calories coming from CHOs are not processed by your body in the same way as calories coming from protein and fat. Your body actually burns about 20 to 25 percent of the calories contained in the CHOs you eat simply to digest them. In addition, CHOs actually can increase your BMR, because they crank up your thyroid hormones, which, in turn, increase your metabolism. This is referred to as the *negative caloric effect* of CHOs. By contrast, only about 3 to 5 percent of the calories in dietary fat are used up in digestion, so the net result is that 100 calories coming from CHO promote far less weight gain than 100 calories coming from fat.

WHAT WE SHOULD EAT—THE BASIC BREAKDOWN

The vast majority of nutritionists recommend that 60 percent of our total calories come from complex CHOs (starches, potatoes, pasta, rice, beans, and most fruits and vegetables), 10 to 15 percent from proteins, and that 25 to 30 percent of our total calories come from fat (with no more than one-third of it being in the form of "saturated" fat—animal fat that is solid at room temperature).

But recent information regarding the relationship between CHO intake and insulin release suggests that we revise our optimum CHO intake downward. It seems that when certain types of CHO are eaten and then digested in the intestine, glucose is released from the CHO and absorbed too quickly. This in turn causes a rapid, sustained release of insulin from the pancreas, which has the direct adverse effects we've already discussed. On top of this, it may also promote the manufacture and storage of excess body fat. For this reason, several studies, including two published in 1997 in the *Journal of the American Medical Association* and the *American Journal of Clinical Nutrition,* recommend that for maximal health, we should probably be getting *only 40 to 50 percent of our total calories from CHO.* In addition, we should make an effort to maximize our intake of low-glycemic-index CHOs (CHOs that are more slowly broken down into glucose in the intestine, like fruits and vegetables, including beans), and minimize our intake of high-glycemic-intake CHOs (quick conversion to glucose) like rice and pasta, which promote the rapid, sustained release of insulin.

This new information has made me switch to aiming for getting only *50 percent of my total dietary calories in the form of CHOs,* and to maximizing the amount of this CHO that comes from fruits and vegetables, including legumes. However, this means I now have to make up for the 10 percent of my total daily calories I am no longer getting in CHO, either in increased dietary protein, fat, or a little of both. My inclination is to *increase protein intake from 10 percent to 20 percent* of my total calories and to try to get at least half of that protein in the form of soybean protein (for reasons discussed below).

There is one other issue we need to consider here, the "biological value" of protein. There are essentially twenty different amino acids that our bodies require to make protein, only nine of which are *essential* amino acids—meaning we cannot make them, so we must get them from our diet. Therefore, if you are eating a protein source lacking in one or more of these essential amino acids, you will ultimately become protein deficient. If you eat meat or dairy products, this is not going to happen. But if you are a vegetarian, you need to eat several different kinds of beans (including soybeans) along with the rest of your vegetables to insure you will get all nine of your essential amino acids.

WHAT WE SHOULD EAT—SOME SPECIFICS

Dietary Fiber: You should also pay attention to your dietary fiber. Recommended intakes are around five grams for each 400 calories you consume daily. Fruits and vegetables are high in fiber, or you can purchase various types of fiber at your drugstore, and add it to your food. This may be one of the most important ways you can prevent colon cancer, a common and fatal cancer in the United States.

Cholesterol: We need some cholesterol to live (it's part of our cell membranes), so most authorities say to limit our intake to less than 300 milligrams a day. However, since our livers make cholesterol, many nutritionists recommend a zero daily cholesterol intake. Cholesterol is only found in animal products, so to avoid cholesterol completely, you must avoid animal products completely, including most dairy products.

DIETARY CHANGES TO AID IN CHOLESTEROL REDUCTION

Soybeans: In addition to decreasing foods high in cholesterol and saturated fat (which the liver converts to cholesterol), you should

171

CHOLESTEROL: THE GOAL OF 150 AND 3:1

What should your cholesterol numbers be? The American Heart Association and National Cholesterol Education Program guidelines say that most people should reduce their total cholesterol to 200 or less, their LDL cholesterol to 130 or less, and keep their total cholesterol to HDL-cholesterol ratio at 5:1 or less.

But several recent studies suggest we need to be more stringent with our goals. In the famous Framingham Heart Study, it was found that a ratio of total cholesterol to HDL cholesterol of 5:1 put you at *average* risk for developing heart disease in this country; but you need to remember that the average American eventually gets heart disease. This study found that you are much better off getting your ratio down to 4:1, and getting it down to 3:1 would be absolutely ideal. However, for most people this requires regular exercising, and removing all cholesterol from one's diet—which basically means completely eliminating all meat and dairy products.

The Framingham Heart Study also found that people with total cholesterol levels of around 200 get heart disease all the time. What we really need to do is get our total cholesterol levels down as close to 150 as possible, because at this level, heart disease is practically nonexistent.

Numerous clinical studies have recently concluded that people who are unable to lower their total cholesterol levels to below 200 with exercise and diet should talk to their physicians about using cholesterol-lowering "statin" drugs. These drugs have now been shown to significantly decrease the risk of a first heart attack in people who currently have no detectable heart disease.

try increasing your soybean intake. Lowered cholesterol levels are a consistent finding in studies of soybean diets, making the regular use of soybeans an important way to increase your Youthspan. Until I began reading the impressive literature on the potential health benefits of this bean, I was not a big fan of it, but several new soy products, including different types of tofu, soyburgers, and soybean "sausages," have made it easier for me to make soybeans a regular part of my diet.

Garlic: Garlic, like soybeans, absolutely lowers cholesterol—and there is a lot of science to prove it. Various types of cholesterol-lowering drugs are available, but before discussing their possible use with your doctor, I strongly recommend a diet low in saturated fats and cholesterol, and high in soybeans and garlic, along with exercise. The effect is similar to anticholesterol drugs, but without the expense and the side effects. If this type of diet does not get your total cholesterol down into the 150 range, then consider the use of cholesterol-lowering drugs.

Sodium: In addition to cholesterol, another common dietary constituent that needs to be controlled is sodium. Limit your sodium intake to less than 2,400 milligrams a day (around 1 teaspoon.) Although essential to good health, sodium has many potential adverse effects, not the least of which is that it can produce hypertension in some people if consumed chronically. However, if you are one of those people who think liberally using the salt shaker is okay because high sodium intakes don't increase your blood pressure (i.e., when it comes to blood pressure, you are "sodium insensitive"), you might want to think again. Recent animal studies now show that high sodium intake greatly increases the incidence of stroke, even when it produces no changes in blood pressure at all. Canned foods such as soups, as well as preserved foods of all types, tend to be very high in sodium. Look for the "low-sodium" alternatives.

Dietary Fat: I told you previously that only 25 to 30 percent of our total calories each day should come from fat, with only one-third of this in the form of saturated fat. Although we have been brainwashed to believe that all fat is bad, this is simply not the case. It is saturated fat, because of it's chemical composition, that is readily converted to cholesterol by our bodies, and it is this fat that should be avoided.

There are two things that you should begin doing right now (in addition to decreasing your saturated fat intake) that will go a long way over the years to increasing your Youthspan. First, you need to stop eating and cooking with margarines, especially "hard" margarines, and shortenings! These contain partially hydrogenated vegetable oils, which form substances known as "trans fatty acids" (TFAs). All you need to know about TFAs is that they increase your cholesterol levels, and thus your risk of heart disease. Many baked goods (such as cookies) contain TFAs as well. If partially hydrogenated vegetable oil is on the list of ingredients, avoid it.

Finally, start cooking with olive oil or canola oil. These oils are now known to be much healthier for your heart than other oils, for many reasons. If you follow these simple rules, your cardiovascular system will thank you.

Dietary Iron and Your Health

Iron is one of those minerals that most people believe you can't get enough of. In the past, the emphasis in many countries, including the United States, was preventing iron-deficiency anemia, so many foods were fortified with iron. In fact, we still tend to view getting loads of iron as a good thing; foods labeled "fortified with iron" apparently remain attractive to many consumers.

We certainly need some iron in our diets to prevent anemia and to supply the enzymes in our cells that need it to work properly. And some people need iron more than others, including growing children and menstruating and pregnant women. But there appear to be some disastrous consequences of having too much iron in our diets, particularly in older adults. To understand these, we need to know a little about how our body absorbs and stores this mineral.

The iron in our diet comes in basically two forms, "heme" iron from meat, and "nonheme" iron from plants. When our bodies have sufficient iron from the latter source, they stop absorbing more iron; but there is no efficient mechanism for limiting the amount of heme iron our intestines absorb. Once we do absorb iron in any form, our bodies tend to hold on to it by storing it in our blood and tissues, and that is where the trouble begins. Recall the "Fenton reaction" in which iron reacts with hydrogen peroxide in cells and forms the ever dangerous hydroxyl radicals. This means that excess stores of iron lead to excess generation of free radicals, which, in turn, lead to an increased incidence of age-related diseases.

A number of studies bear out this danger of too much iron in our diets, especially if that iron comes from an animal source. In one study of almost 2,000 Finnish men, it was shown that those men with the highest blood-iron reserves were more than twice as likely to suffer from coronary heart disease as those men with lower levels. And in a long-term study of 14,000 adults, those with the highest levels of stored iron were found to be more likely to develop cancer, particularly if they were men.

Fortunately, there are tests to find out if you have too much iron in your body. The most reliable of these is the serum ferritin test; if your serum ferritin levels are greater than 200, you need to think about decreasing your iron stores.

The simplest way to do this is to start eating more vegetables and less meat. Another thing you need to do is donate blood every sixty days until your serum ferritin levels are in an acceptable range. Also, if you take vitamin-C supplements, you should cut back to 250 milligrams a day, either three hours before or after a meal, as this vitamin is particularly efficient at increasing intestinal absorption of nonheme iron. Finally, it is interesting to note that a study published in the journal *Heart* in September of 1997 found that people who had not given blood in the past were almost twice as likely to have had a heart attack or stroke as people who had donated blood. It was suggested that the reason for this may be due to the expected lower iron stores in blood donors. So now you have two good reasons to donate blood—you could be saving your own life, as well as someone else's.

PART VI

✵

FEELING YOUNG AND SEXY

*Y*outh implies a long list of capabilities: strength, vitality, mental sharpness, healthiness, resilience. But when you ask someone in her seventies or eighties what youth is, above all she will say that youth is a *feeling*.

"It's a feeling you wake up with and go to sleep with," one woman in her midseventies explained to me. "And you can't say exactly what it is until it isn't there any more."

Happily, the Youthspan-extending tools that are available to us today go a very long way, both directly and indirectly, chemically and psychologically, in promoting that quintessential youthful feeling, one variously described to me as "hopefulness," "feeling full of life," "happy," "peppy," and—a word that I hear with surprising frequency—"sexy."

"Sure, sexy," one woman in her late sixties told me. "When you are young, you go through each day looking at the men who pass your way through special eyes—the eyes of a woman who enjoys a man's manliness. And when you no longer examine the goods that way, you know you are over the hill. All the rest of the bad feelings that come with advanced age—the depression, the hopelessness—follow from that one."

Although this woman may be overstating the case a bit, there is no doubt in my mind that age-associated depression is often intimately connected to a waning libido and/or sexual dysfunction, such as impotence. This connection is both psychological and biochemical. For starters, a sexually alive and active person feels good about himself because he still has the fundamental passion and power of youth. And the biochemical fact is that those same major hormone supplements that can potentially revitalize sexual feelings—DHEA, testosterone, and estrogen—also have been shown to reverse age-associated depression on their own, when used properly.

The connection between libido and general mood is particularly relevant during what we call early middle age, our forties and fifties. I can vouch for this from all the nervous gags about "down time" that I hear at my over-thirty basketball games.

IF YOU REALLY WANT TO GET DEPRESSED, TAKE AN ANTIDEPRESSANT

These days, middle-aged men and women with sagging energy, spirits, and self-esteem are routinely diagnosed with low-grade depression and put on one of the new menu of antidepressants with few side effects like Prozac, Desipramine, and Zoloft. Unfortunately, one side effect that remains in a significant number of cases is sexual dysfunction in the form of radically reduced libido, an inability to reach orgasm, or impotence. Hey, but at least you're not depressed, right?

Wrong. A woman with a sagging libido is a woman who feels her best days are behind her. And a man who cannot get an erection is undoubtedly a seriously depressed man.

To my mind, any doctor faced with a depressed middle-aged patient should prescribe moderate exercise, as well as take assays of that person's DHEA, testosterone, and/or estrogen to determine if they are present in *youthful* amounts before even thinking of prescribing an antidepressant. Not only can exercise, as well as replenishing these hormones to youthful levels directly enhance mood, they can indirectly do the job by increasing sexual desire and sexual energy, quite the opposite from the effects of a "legitimate" antidepressant.

WORTS AND ALL

Another route worth considering is St. John's wort, a perennial shrub (also know as *Hypericum perforatum*) that had been pretty much dismissed by the American medical community until a 1996 study in the *British Medical Journal* that analyzed twenty-three human trials involving over 1,700 depressed patients. The conclusion was that the herb worked just as well as standard antidepressants, while causing *far fewer side effects,* and costing only around twenty-five cents a day. Not good news for the multimillion-dollar pharmaceutical market for synthetic antidepressant drugs. The optimum dose seems to be around 300 milligrams of St. John's wort extract, containing 0.3 percent hypericum, taken three times a day. However, it can take four to six weeks to begin working. Be absolutely sure you do not mix it with any other antidepressants you might be taking.

CHAPTER THIRTEEN

Young and Sexy Tools I:
Hormones

From the time we were teenagers and our parents cautioned us about our "raging hormones," we have known that hormones and sex were intimately related. Although I discussed the hormones DHEA, growth hormone, and melatonin under "Muscle and Energy Tools," all three of these hormones can contribute to our sexual feelings; similarly, although the hormones estrogen and testosterone have a marked effect on our sexuality and mood, they have substantial effects in many other areas too.

Estrogen

WHAT IT IS AND HOW IT WORKS

Not only does estrogen increase the lifespan of the postmenopausal women who take it, it enhances their Youthspan, allowing them to live with a much higher quality of life. Estrogen hormone-replacement therapy (EHRT) prevents women from suffering from the infamous "hot flashes," vaginal dryness, and night sweats associated with postmenopausal loss of estrogen. And, of course, EHRT often significantly enhances a woman's postmenopausal libido. But even more importantly, EHRT provides a significant reduction in the risk for cardiovascular disease, stroke, and osteoporosis.

Women who have not reached menopause suffer fewer heart attacks than men their age, but we now know this difference is largely due to premenopausal women's higher levels of estrogen; once they do reach menopause and experience estrogen decline, their risk of heart attack climbs up until it is the same or even greater than men's—that is, unless these women are undergoing EHRT.

Estrogen keeps total blood-cholesterol levels down and raises the blood levels of HDL, which helps explain why EHRT cuts the risk for heart disease. Also, it has been found that this hormone can act as a potent free-radical scavenger; this means that it might be important in blocking free-radical oxidation of LDL, the kind of cholesterol that can cause your coronary arteries to clog up fast. And EHRT now appears to make another tremendous contribution to a woman's Youthspan; several recent studies have shown that it may prevent or delay the onset of Alzheimer's disease.

On top of all this, EHRT has a clear cosmetic effect by promoting moist, unwrinkled skin. A 1997 study of nearly 4,000 postmenopausal women found that those using EHRT were significantly less likely to have dry or wrinkled skin than those not using it. One reason for this appears to be estrogen's ability to preserve the collagen content of skin (the "cement" that holds your skin cells in place).

Sadly, more than half of the postmenopausal women in this country do not use EHRT. One of the reasons for this is that although many of them have heard about the risks of EHRT (slight increase in the risk of breast cancer and endometrial cancer, the tissue lining the uterus), women do not know much about the potential benefits of EHRT. It has been shown in some studies that one of the major reasons for this is that their doctors simply do not tell them about these benefits. Amazingly, two fairly recent studies have shown that this is due to the fact that the physicians themselves simply do not know enough about EHRT to give their patients good advice about it. And if most physicians do not keep up with the extensive scientific literature on EHRT, it would certainly be hard to count on them to be familiar with scientific literature about replacement therapy with GH, DHEA, or testosterone.

Although the slight increase in risk of breast cancer is real in women using EHRT, the decision to forego EHRT may still be due to the inaccurate way that EHRT/breast-cancer studies are presented to the public. For example, the 1995 Colditz study reported that there was a 45 percent increase in the risk of breast cancer in women who were on EHRT for ten or more years. But what exactly does this mean—that forty-five out of a hundred will develop breast cancer if they are on EHRT for more than ten years? No way. A better way to understand these potentially misleading statistics is as follows:

If one hundred women who were fifty years old and *not* using EHRT were followed for twenty years, epidemiological evidence shows that about five of those women would develop breast cancer. If those same women lived another ten years to age eighty, three more (a total of eight out of a hundred) would get breast cancer. Now, if these same women had been receiving EHRT alone (without any progestin), epidemiological evidence shows that an additional two women would have gotten breast cancer by age seventy; and if these women lived to age eighty, another two would have gotten breast cancer; that is, a total of twelve out of a hundred, instead of the eight out of one hundred women who did *not* use EHRT.

This is certainly a real risk, but most would consider it an *acceptable* risk given the fact that those women who did not use EHRT would have been much more likely to acquire osteoporosis, heart disease, or suffer a stroke long before age eighty. Not to mention the fact that they would have had to live that time with chronic vaginal problems, hot flashes, and night sweats. *The reality is that heart disease kills many more postmenopausal women than does breast cancer.*

Obviously, the decision to use EHRT is between you and your physician. It needs to be based on a number of factors, including any predisposing risk factors you may have for breast cancer. However, if you are a woman reaching or have already reached menopause, but are not using EHRT, I strongly advise you to read up on the scientific literature to help you make your decision; and make sure also that your physician is well educated about EHRT, because it is your health that is on the line here.

DOSAGE

Your physician needs to determine the dose of estrogen that is specifically best for you. It is equally important that you and your doctor carefully consider what type of estrogen is best for you. Premarin, the most commonly prescribed form of oral estrogen, is actually a myriad of estrogens found in the urine of pregnant horses; it only contains tiny amounts of estradiol, the most potent form of natural estrogen in the human body, and it also includes many foreign estrogens. Fortunately, synthetic estradiol is also now available; it can be taken in pill form, as a skin patch, or as a vaginal cream. And there is currently a move in research circles to produce "smart" estrogens (called SERMs) that could produce the same benefits as the current estrogens used in EHRT, but would not cause an increased risk of breast cancer. In fact, the first SERM, the Eli Lily drug "Raloxifene," was approved by the FDA in late 1997 and should be available in early 1998. Ask your physician about the advantages and disadvantages of this compound, which has been dubbed "estrogen light."

Finally, if EHRT is not doing the job on your libido that you had hoped it would, many endocrinologists are now suggesting to postmenopausal women that some testosterone be given along with estrogen. Discuss this with a knowledgeable physician.

Testosterone

WHAT IT IS AND HOW IT WORKS

Few honest men over fifty will deny that their interest in sex has become significantly lower than it was at, say, twenty-five. For a while there, the psychologists and sexologists of America were trying mightily to convince us that this decline was "all in our heads"— that our libido was only flagging because we thought it was. Testosterone-replacement therapy suggests otherwise.

Sexual function has two major components in men: desire, which centers around the brain; and the actual physical ability to produce an erection, which involves a number of body systems, including the brain, but also the blood vessels and the autonomic nervous system. Testosterone is associated with the psychological component of erection—a testosterone deficiency is definitely correlated with a psychological loss of desire for sex. Several studies have shown a clear correlation between declining plasma levels of testosterone and declining sexual desire; several others have demonstrated that this lack of sexual desire usually improves greatly if the men are given testosterone supplements. Dr. Edward Klaiber, an endocrinologist at the Worcester Foundation for Biomedical Research in Shrewsbury, Massachusetts, has used testosterone to treat impotence in dozens of older men, and claims 80 percent of these patients have been pleased with the results.

Of course, if you are one of those older men who still has a desire for sex, but is unable to achieve an erection because of a physiological problem such as hypertension, atherosclerosis, or diabetes, testosterone will *not* help you. Fortunately, there are other treatments that can alleviate these problems. Therefore, if you are experiencing erratic erections or impotence, it is very important to see your doctor. Find out if it is due to loss of libido, which testosterone supplementation can usually remedy, or an underlying physiological problem, which other treatments can.

But the question of impotence aside, an increased libido has major implications for every middle-aged man: When we feel more sexually alert and more easily aroused, we feel young in ways that cannot be measured. Males receiving testosterone-replacement therapy often say that they have more energy. One of the reasons for this is that this hormone increases the number of red blood cells (RBCs) in our blood (males often experience a gradual decline in RBCs as they age).

As a lecturer at our medical school on reproductive hormones, I have often wondered what kind of "sexism" accounts for the fact that testosterone-replacement therapy for men has lagged so far behind estrogen-replacement therapy for women. Could it be because male researchers were somehow loath to acknowledge the age-related decline of this quintessential "macho" hormone?

Whatever the reason, for more than forty years researchers have understood the benefits of treating women with estrogen supplements when their ovaries fail during menopause, but did not seriously look at the possibility of giving middle-aged men testosterone supplementation to compensate for the decline in output of this hormone by their aging testes until the last decade. In fact, it is only very recently that the public at large has been exposed to the fact that a lack of testosterone contributes mightily to the aging process in males.

One nonpsychological reason for the discrepancy between research on estrogen replacement and research on testosterone replacement is that the drop in estrogen in women is quite rapid. This occurs over just a couple of years and results in rapid onset of estrogen-deficiency symptoms, while the loss of testosterone in men is more gradual. There is a considerable amount of variability among individual men in relation to how much testosterone levels actually decline with age, but testosterone can drop as much as 40 percent between the ages of forty and seventy. And it may take ten or more years after age forty-five before a man starts to show the classic symptoms of testosterone deficiency. These are a decrease in muscle mass, an increase in body fat, lack of energy, declining interest in sex, depression and feelings of worthlessness, cognitive impairment, and brittle bones due to osteoporosis. In fact, many scientists now refer to the more gradual drop in testosterone in men as the "male menopause" or "andropause."

Just how much does this testosterone drop affect the middle-aged male's Youthspan? Much more than you undoubtedly imagined. Consider the consequences of supplementing testosterone in middle-aged men on their body fat, muscle mass and strength, and bone density. Most men over fifty are well aware of the fact that they have more body fat and less muscle than they did when they were twenty; if not, most are reminded of it every time they look in the mirror. Well, it turns out that it is not simply middle-aged sloth that accounts for this. Dr. Joyce Tenover, a gerontology researcher at the University of Washington in Seattle, demonstrated in 1992 that weekly injections of testosterone for three months in a test group of middle-aged men resulted in a significant increase in lean body mass and a decrease in bone reabsorption (a cause of fragile bones).

Subsequent studies have corroborated her results. Dr. John Morley, a gerontology researcher at the St. Louis University School of Medicine, showed that three months of testosterone therapy significantly increased muscle strength in men over seventy. In another recent study, a group of men in their sixties receiving testosterone injections developed significant increases in leg muscle strength. Incidently, these test subjects also experienced a decrease in the amount of total and LDL cholesterol.

Of course, like anything else, too much of a good thing can be a problem. If you take too much testosterone and therefore produce too many RBCs, your blood can literally become too "thick" and you could end up having a stroke. However, simply monitoring your hematocrit and regulating your testosterone intake will completely mitigate against this eventuality.

Dr. Morley believes that age-related testosterone loss may play a significant role in age-related memory dysfunction. At the annual meeting of the Endocrine Society in 1994, Dr. Morley showed data from an ongoing study of men over fifty which demonstrated that during the first six months of the process, testosterone therapy markedly improved performance on memory tests. In addition, multiple studies have shown that younger men perform better on tasks of spatial cognition—visual perception, spatial attention, object identification, and visual memory processes—than older men. Now researchers have shown that older men receiving testosterone therapy for three months experienced a significant improvement in spatial cognition.

We also now know that testosterone has a profound effect on mood, and can therefore be important in preventing one of the most common Youthspan abbreviators: depression. Many clinical studies have demonstrated that depressed people tend to have lower blood levels of testosterone and that people on testosterone-replacement therapy report an increased sense of well-being. And obviously, there is a strong positive correspondence between increased libido and an increased sense of well-being.

DOSAGE

If you are a male over fifty years old, and believe that you may need testosterone-hormone-replacement therapy (THRT), you should seek out a knowledgeable physician and have your levels of total and free testosterone measured. Again, you will want to determine how your plasma levels compare to an average man of twenty-five, not to other males your age who undoubtedly also have experienced a decline in biologically active testosterone.

One of the reasons some physicians may balk at giving you THRT, even if your levels of bioavailable testosterone are quite low, is that they are afraid you will develop benign prostatic hypertrophy (an enlarged prostate gland), or even prostate cancer. In fact, there is no compelling evidence that THRT causes benign prostatic hypertrophy or prostate cancer, only evidence that if you already have these disorders, THRT may make them worse. This is why if you are considering THRT, you must have a complete blood chemistry done that includes a hematocrit, a digital prostate exam, and a prostate specific antigen (PSA) blood test.

If you and your doctor decide to start you on a testosterone regime, you should continue to monitor your hematocrit, PSA, and prostate size every few months to see if there are any adverse changes. If your PSA or hematocrit rises significantly, and/or your prostate enlarges, you need to cut back the dose of testosterone. If the problems fail to resolve, you need to cut back even further, or consider stopping the use of THRT altogether.

Another unfounded fear is that THRT increases the risk of heart disease in men. The reality is that while some synthetic versions of testosterone raise blood levels of LDL cholesterol and lower levels of HDL cholesterol, natural testosterone itself does not seem to adversely affect plasma-cholesterol profiles. Thus, the bottom line is that most older men can find a level of THRT that is safe and effective.

One last point: As of quite recently, it is no longer necessary to inject synthetic testosterone or testosterone-like drugs into muscle. The FDA has approved a testosterone patch with the brand name Androderm that releases natural testosterone in levels that mimic the body's own release of testosterone, bringing levels up to those seen in young men. This user-friendly form of testosterone is a welcome arrival, as only about 250,000 of the estimated four to five million men in the United States alone with testosterone deficiency (most of it age-related) actually receive THRT.

ALTERNATIVES TO THRT

Testosterone can be transformed into estradiol by enzymes in fat cells; therefore, overweight older men may be making plenty of testosterone but have lower than normal testosterone levels because their fat cells are converting too much of it to estrogen. So, if your doctor determines that your free and total plasma-testosterone levels are much lower than they should be *and* you are overweight, simply losing weight should be tried before using THRT.

Finally, DHEA supplements often increase testosterone levels, so if you are using DHEA, and a comparison of pre- and post-DHEA blood tests reveals that you are one of those men who readily converts some DHEA to testosterone, taking DHEA may obviate any need you will ever have for THRT.

CHAPTER FOURTEEN

Young and Sexy Tools II: Changing Your Mindset

An elder who has the mind and vigor of a young person is in possession of the best of both worlds: knowledge based on experience combined with the ability to access, analyze, and articulate that knowledge. But accepting both of these worlds proves more troublesome than you might expect. We have to overcome a mindset that posits the attributes of youth and advanced age in opposing categories, each with a long list of mutually exclusive characteristics—a list that says you cannot be both full of stamina *and* full of wisdom; you cannot be both quick witted *and* have a deep philosophical perspective; you cannot have both boundless energy and the good sense to stop and smell the roses.

Wrong! With the advent of new medical discoveries, we are certainly capable of combining these traditional opposites. But in order to exploit these remarkable new youth extenders, we must first abandon these limiting mindsets. This means letting go of long-held beliefs such as the popular notion that we should learn to grow old gracefully. Roughly translated, this expression means: Give in to the inevitable and do it without complaining. (The inevitable, of course, is increasing forgetfulness, loss of zest for life, and general ill health.) Like most bromides, this one is intended to guard us against pain and disappointment—if we gracefully accept the inevitable, it won't hurt so much.

But something else happens when we gracefully accept the inevitable and that is that we unwittingly make it happen. It becomes a self-fulfilling prophecy: feeble and forgetful we are if we think we are. Like so much else in mind-body rotary traffic, negative signals from the mind result in physical handicaps which, in turn, promote more mental negativity.

In her seminal work on brain fitness, the French psychologist, Monique Le Poncin, asserts, "It is not because some of their neurons become quiescent and gaps appear in their memories that older people . . . behave as if they had been defeated in life. The opposite is true: it is because they are psychologically weak . . . and lose their motivation that regions of their brain eventually become quiescent."

Guided Imagery

"The imagination is probably a person's least utilized health resource," says Martin Rossman, M.D., cofounder of the Academy for Guided Imagery. We all know that our imaginations can have an immediate impact on our bodies; anyone who has ever had a sexual fantasy knows that. But undoubtedly, our most common imaginings are those personal scenarios with disastrous endings known as worries. And worrying has the impact on our bodies of making it less resistant to infection and disease. Happily, according to Rossman, "the people who worry the most are the ones most likely to benefit the most from effective guided imagery, as the process of worrying yourself sick and imagining yourself well are very similar."

Like meditation and biofeedback, guided imagery can help us remain healthy and young by directly affecting physiological processes in a positive direction—including heart rate, blood pressure, hormone levels, and immune function. But it can also benefit us by leading us to insights into our health and body functions, and by elevating our mood.

Visualizing a Long Youthspan

One of the most effective ways to change a mindset is through visualization—creating a new image in your mind and exploring and playing with it for a few minutes each day. If you regularly try this technique, you will soon find that you have transformed this image into a new perspective that stays with you throughout your day, replacing the mindset that has been limiting your perspective and your possibilities. In effect, what you will have done is a little brain recircuiting, willfully changing sets of neural pathways, thus creating new mental associations. For us, that means setting up an entirely new way of visualizing moving through our forties, fifties, sixties, seventies, and beyond—of making the very idea of a long Youthspan a reasonable expectation instead of a contradiction in terms.

Let us start by visualizing a reconciliation of one of these so-called contradictions I mentioned above—the one that asserts you cannot be both full of stamina and full of wisdom.

Visualization Exercise I

WISE MAN ON THE FOUL LINE

Sitting quietly with your eyes closed, imagine yourself as a man or woman of seventy-five. Your teenage grandson is visiting and tells you about a problem he is having at school with one of his teachers. You reach back sixty years and tell him a parallel story or two from your own past, adding the perspective of how you see the incident now. Old-fashioned grandfatherly wisdom, right?

But now, with your grandson feeling better after your chat, you suggest that the two of you go outside and toss a few hoops—maybe a game of O-U-T. At first, the image seems almost comical, doesn't it? The wise old man can't play basketball too, can he?

Yup, he can. There is no implicit contradiction here. Stick with the image. Shoot a few hoops, joke around, go inside for a Coke.

I guarantee that you will come out of this little mental scenario smiling. Try it again another day, say, while you are sitting on the train or even waiting at a stop light (eyes open this time, however). Soon you will feel comfortable with this image—the transformation from image to possibility to expectation has begun. And along with this mental transformation comes a physical transformation that reaches right into your nervous and immune systems, making them more available to the therapies and supplements that extend your Youthspan.

Obviously, you can create your own scripts for your visualizations. A good way to start is to identify some assumption that you have been carrying around about the inevitable consequences of aging, and then create a scenario that turns it around. Say you are convinced that you will lose your memory—in fact, that you have already begun to lose your memory. Construct a scenario in which your memory is sharp, where you have phone numbers at your finger tips and can recall whole passages of books you read long ago. Imagine really being such a person with these capabilities. Explore it, play with it, make it a personal possibility.

Visualization Exercise II

HORMONAL TOUR

Sitting quietly with your eyes closed, imagine a DHEA molecule working its way through your body. Visualize it like a Jules Verne voyage—watch the molecule swimming in your bloodstream.

As it wends its way, everything it touches comes alive. Cells brighten like flowers touched by a summer rain. Now it contacts your muscles and the tissue pulses with new energy. Excess fat melts, your skin tightens. Now the DHEA molecule sails up your spine into your central nervous system to your brain. Your brain starts to crackle and glow like an engine that has suddenly been fed high-test fuel. Synapses flash like lightning bolts. Your whole body and mind vibrate with smooth energy.

Does such a visualization fantasy actually make any difference in the way our bodies are affected by the infusion of DHEA as some mind/body healers claim? Or is it just a silly New Age mind game that has nothing to do with our body chemistry? This debate rages on with new studies coming in daily, including data from psychoneuroimmunologists.

But from my perspective, there is good reason to try such visualization exercises however that debate is resolved. And that is because the exercise makes us mindful of whatever changes the DHEA (or other medication/supplement) creates. In other words, even if the visualization does not contribute at the biochemical level to making the supplement more effective at, say, providing us with more energy, it does increase our consciousness of whatever new energy the DHEA on its own makes available to us. And there is a very definite sense in which this consciousness is necessary for using and enjoying that newly available energy.

One final visualization . . .

Visualization Exercise III

MAGIC MIRROR

Sitting quietly with your eyes closed, imagine waking up one morning feeling younger by ten years. See yourself bounding out of bed and going to the bathroom mirror. Sure enough, there is definitely something different about the appearance of your face. You see it first in your eyes—they seem brighter, more alert, less troubled. But it's in the muscle tone of your face, too—you look more relaxed, less anxious, more alive. You think about your day and you find yourself eager to get it started. You've got lots to do but energy to spare.

Then it dawns on you: it has actually started to happen—you are getting younger! And you know in your heart that this is just the beginning. Your biological clock is running in reverse!

I can hear the skeptics more loudly this time. Yeah, sure, this visualization stuff works, because all it really amounts to is self-delusion. It's a way of pulling the wool over your own eyes. You convince yourself you are growing younger, so you don't see the wrinkles. It's like the bald guy who tilts his head when he looks in the mirror so he can delude himself into thinking he has a full head of hair.

To which I can only reply: Maybe the real delusion is that you really are growing older, and the Triple-Your-Youthspan Program is having no effect on how you age.

My point is more than, Young you are if you think you are—although there is an element of truth in that, too. Rather it is the well-documented psychological fact that expectations influence responses. For example, if you expect to remember a telephone number, there is a much greater likelihood that you will remember the number than if you do not expect to remember it. Ditto for energy, reflexes, perceptual acuity, even weight loss.

Another way you can set up this psychological phenomenon for yourself is by acting younger around other people. Even if at first there is an element of pretense in this act, it will soon become self-fulfilling. Part of the reason for this is that when people respond to you as if you are younger than you are, you feel younger and so act younger. Round and round it goes, and you feel younger with each revolution. So here is one hint for getting this youth-promoting mental cycle going: Stop joking about growing old all the time! Yes, I know these gags are a staple of my over-thirty basketball team, but they really do not help you feel younger.

PART VII

🍂

HEY, GOOD-LOOKING!

"I want to die young so I'll have a good-looking corpse," Mark Twain said, mocking one of our greatest fears about aging. Second only to our fear of *feeling* old is our fear of *looking* old. But fortunately, we again find ourselves in possession of a variety of effective tools available for preserving a good-looking face and figure well into what used to be called old age—and I am not talking about cosmetic surgery.

The aspect of our appearance that is perhaps most vulnerable to age and most alarmingly visible is our skin. Skin can wrinkle, discolor, and sag with the passage of time. Yet just because you are becoming older doesn't mean you have to acquire wrinkled skin. But you need to get started early on this one, folks, because damage to skin accumulates over years—when the damage reaches a critical stage, you suddenly find yourself with wrinkled skin, lookin' old.

There are three subtle aspects of our appearance that benefit a great deal from Youthspan tools: the good health, high energy, and intelligence that we project, particularly from our faces and eyes. When vigor and vitality radiate from our skin and eyes, we definitely look attractive and youthful to the people around us—especially in contrast to those people who appear perpetually on the verge of some illness or infection and those people who are constantly tired. And when we radiate alertness and intelligence, we find heads turning in our direction—any beauty maven will tell you that the bright eyes and engaged, expressive face of an active mind are ultimately as important as a well-turned ankle.

Needless to say, looking good is a great tonic to our disposition, and that goes for men as well as women. We all know that when we make a good visual impression on other people, their responses are the best mirrors we can ever have. And even if our hair is gray or thinning, as long as our bodies are erect and vital, our muscles well toned, and our skin firm, thick, and smooth, we retain an overall youthful appearance.

REUNION REVISITED

Let us hearken back to that college reunion I alluded to earlier, the spectacle of Joe Canty, once captain of our soccer team, now looking seriously old, wrinkled, and decrepit, compared with the phenomenon of Bob Corey, his eyes clear, his skin tight and un-wrinkled, his figure slim and erect, his gait brisk and confident. The temptation was to chalk up the difference between the two of them to fate in the form of genetics. But after speaking with each of them, I drew a very different conclusion.

Joe had encountered what he considered some bad luck in the form of a bout with skin cancer and a long series of infectious diseases. Indeed, both of these were extremely unfortunate and had taken their highly visible toll on his appearance. But I was unwilling to chalk it all up to bad luck because Joe had not played the odds well, to say the least: he had been a heavy smoker, he had lain out in the sun unprotected every summer and winter vacation; he had never exercised or watched his diet; he never hedged his bet against wrinkled skin and infectious diseases with antioxidants; and he never had his hormone levels checked and possibly corrected when he reached his forties.

Bob, on the other hand, had taken good care of himself in every way that Joe had not. This is surely the most anecdotal of evidence, but the difference was right there in front of my eyes: Joe looked old and unattractive, Bob looked youthful and attractive.

CHAPTER FIFTEEN

Looking Good Tools I: Skin Don'ts

Our skin is our first line of defense against all invaders. It basically comes in two layers: the outer "epidermal" layer and the inner "dermal" layer. It is the dermal layer that provides most of the support for nice, taut skin, thanks mostly to the dermal proteins collagen and elastin. Once these proteins are destroyed in sufficient amounts, there is no turning back—the damage is irreversible (although Retin-A seems to offer some benefits to already damaged skin).

Dermatologists will tell you that the most tried-and-true therapy for keeping your skin young is to simply stay out of direct sunlight as much as possible; that tan you long for now will be a major reason why your skin will wrinkle before its time. And I'm not talking about just limiting the time you spend on the beach. Most of the sun damage that accumulates over the years in our skin comes from the daily exposure we get just walking down the street, working in the yard, or waiting for a taxi.

Most of the sunlight that damages our skin is the ultraviolet "B" waves (UVB), which are partially screened out by the ozone layer, but still make it to the earth's surface in large amounts (UVA rays are also damaging to the skin, but much less so than UVB rays). Note that these UVB rays are not completely blocked out by clouds, so if you spend a lot of time outside in the summer on cloudy days wearing little clothing, you are putting yourself at risk for early wrinkling of your skin. The ubiquity of UVB rays is the reason why our skin wrinkles at varying rates. The skin that is most commonly exposed to the sun year in and out—our face and arms—is the skin that wrinkles first.

Routine use of sunscreens in the summer (or year round if you live in a tropical climate) not only can prevent skin cancer, but help you prevent skin aging as well. Look for sunscreens that block both UVA and UVB, that have a "sun protection factor" (SPF) of at least 15. The SPF simply indicates the increased amount of time it will take for your skin to burn, compared to using no protection at all. So if you are using a sunscreen with an SPF of 12, it will take twelve times as long for your skin to burn as it would if you weren't using any sunscreen.

The UVB rays can damage our skin cells directly or they can produce oxygen free radicals which will then attack the cell membrane, DNA, and cell proteins of skin cells that make collagen and elastin. Once enough of these cells have been killed, and dermal levels of collagen and elastin drop, skin begins to wrinkle. Because free radicals play such an important role in the development of wrinkled skin, anything else you do that results in excess generation of free radicals will also contribute to skin wrinkling over the years. Cigarette smokers generate lots of excess free radicals in their bodies compared to nonsmokers, so their skin tends to wrinkle much more than that of nonsmokers. Diets high in saturated fats carry lots of calories, which can also result in excess free-radical production. In addition, diets high in polyunsaturated oils (such as vegetable oils) can contribute to wrinkled skin because these oils are taken up into the membranes of skin cells where they are particularly susceptible to attack from free radicals.

CHAPTER SIXTEEN

Looking Good Tools II: Diet and Supplements

Several studies have shown that eating foods high in natural antioxidants like beta carotene protects the skin over the long haul. In fact, at the beginning of this century, doctors used diets high in beta carotene-rich vegetables to protect people with light complexions from sunburn. Similarly, taking beta carotene supplements is a good way to start slowing the process of skin aging. And because free radicals seem to be such major culprits in skin aging, there is good reason to believe that an increased intake of *all* antioxidants would be a natural antidote to skin aging. This may be particularly true for the antioxidant Pycnogenol, because this natural compound has been found to inhibit the enzymes which break down the important skin proteins, collagen and elastin.

Also, estrogen-replacement therapy for postmenopausal women has a demonstrated ability to prevent or slow the winkling and dry skin that we associate with age, yet another reason to use this Youthspan-enhancing hormone therapy.

Retin-A (tretinoin) can significantly slow sun-induced skin aging, and it is currently the only product on the market that may actually undo some of the sun damage to the skin which has already occurred. Retin-A is somewhat similar chemically to the vitamin-A/

beta-carotene family of antioxidants; it works by stimulating cells in the outer layer of the skin to divide, and also seems to produce some collagen growth in the dermal skin layer. However, it can take a long time to produce this effect, and there is only a limited result—if you already have highly damaged skin due to sun damage, don't expect miracles. Retin-A is available only by prescription.

Recently, Dr. Albert Kligman, a dermatologist and professor emeritus at the University of Pennsylvania, stated that beta hydroxy acid (salicylic acid) is about to join alpha hydroxy acid (glycolic acid) as a treatment for aging skin. Salicylic acid has been used by dermatologists for decades to treat acne and other skin problems; now it has been shown to be useful in clearing up fine wrinkles in skin. Dr. Kligman cited a study in which 190 patients applied either salicylic acid, glycolic acid, or a placebo; salicylic acid proved significantly better at improving overall facial appearance, with almost no side effects.

You can buy beta hydroxy acid in drugstores. Dr. Kligman says that when selecting a beta hydroxy acid be sure to look at the product's "pH" (a reflection of how acidic it is). A pH of 4 or 5 renders the product inactive, while a pH that is too low (1) is irritating. He claims a good compromise is a product with a pH of about 3.

PART VIII

WHY YOU HAVE TO BE YOUR OWN BEST ADVOCATE

Drug Money and the Old Boy Network

*T*he Melatonin Secret was out. In popular magazines and television reports, people across the country discovered that a relatively small dose of this inexpensive hormone was not only a safe sleeping potion, but it also held a significant promise for extending our Youthspan. Food-supplement manufacturers could barely keep up with the sudden demand. And making the situation even more fortuitous for the consumer, Congress had recently enacted the new Dietary Supplement Health and Education Act (DSHEA), making a hormone supplement like melatonin readily available without the delay of additional and expensive, time-consuming, product efficacy tests.

And then, on network television, along came a prominent biochemist/physician from a prestigious university with a terrifying melatonin scenario.

"I'm really scared that someone's going to take chronic doses of melatonin for a long time and have all kinds of disturbances in their other biological rhythms, which might lead them to drive into a telephone pole," this good doctor said.

Following up, the NBC correspondent said, "Another fear is that melatonin is sold not as a drug, but as a food supplement like vitamins. A law recently passed by Congress restricts the Food and Drug Administration's ability to regulate food supplements. While there have been no reports of adverse reactions from melatonin, six years ago a manufacturer accidentally contaminated another food supplement used for sleep, called tryptophan, with an unknown toxin. Forty-five people were killed, and hundreds were disabled in this country alone."

Terrifying indeed.

However, one small detail was omitted from this public-interest report: At the time of this broadcast, the diligent university professor (who shall remain nameless) had already obtained a patent for a compound containing melatonin as a prescription sleeping pill, and was in the process of seeking FDA approval to market his version of melatonin through his pharmaceutical company. In other words, if this professor-cum-businessman could get the FDA to classify melatonin as a drug instead of the natural nutritional supplement it was currently deemed, he would be able to corner the market in the entire United States for melatonin-containing sleeping potions—or at the very least, eliminate pure melatonin in the health food store as a competitor for it.

You are probably thinking that the FDA, being an independent federal agency, would not be caught dead granting this professor the status he was seeking for melatonin. I mean, it might have the appearance of something that sounds dangerously like price gouging.

"Don't bet against it," says an individual who is a watchdog of FDA operations. "You'd be surprised just how cozy the FDA is with pharmaceutical companies. It's one of the all-time 'old boy networks.' When policy makers leave the FDA, they usually turn up in executive positions at the very pharmaceutical companies which produce the drugs they have recently approved."

Conspiracy, Conshmeeracy, as Long as You're Healthy

I am not a man given to conspiracy theories. Generally speaking, I do not imagine plots against the ordinary citizen being hatched in high places—or even in low places, for that matter. But over the years that I have been a neuropharmacologist, I have come to believe that not all is as it should be at the Food and Drug Administration. If the FDA's rules and practices are not calculated to put big money in the hands of the major pharmaceutical companies, they are at the very least bent in the direction of depriving ordinary people of the freedom to obtain inexpensive health-and-youth-promoting supplements and nutrients. And that is not good news for those of us who want to Triple Our Youthspan. If melatonin becomes classified as a prescription drug, can other supplements be far behind?

The FDA regulates more than $1 trillion worth of products each year, which is equal to twenty-five cents on every consumer dollar spent in this country. The agency's avowed purpose is to protect the consumer from products that do harm, and from products that they deem inefficacious. These are two very different goals. I certainly don't want to risk ingesting any pill that has a good chance of making me sick or dead. And if anything I take has possible side effects, I want to know exactly what they are, and my chances of incurring them before I swallow it down. Furthermore, if some putative health-enhancing product hasn't a particle of evidence to warrant taking it, I would certainly want access to that information, and exactly how it was arrived at.

But that does not mean I want anyone—government agency or otherwise—to tell me that I can't waste my money on any product if I decide to try it. Of course, I want responsible protection from well-substantiated health risks; but I do not want Big Brother vetting my health-care options. Especially not if Big Brother pals around with people like the aforementioned professor-businessman.

The L-tryptophan Trip-up

Let us go back for a moment to what that reporter had to say about the infamous L-tryptophan incident. This amino acid is a protein building block that was a popular supplement sold in health-food stores and pharmacies from the 1960s until 1989, when it was banned by the FDA. The basic reason for L-tryptophan's popularity was its natural property of increasing production of serotonin, a neurotransmitter that has been shown to promote natural sleep, relieve depression, soothe anxiety and stress, and reduce sensitivity to chronic pain.

Beside insomniacs and depressives, regular users of this supplement included people who suffered from manic-depressive and obsessive-compulsive disorders, and women who suffered from PMS. Because this amino acid is a naturally occurring substance found, for example, in turkey meat and beef, it is unpatentable and relatively inexpensive to produce, thus cheaper by far for the consumer than prescription drugs like Xanax, Valium, Halcion, Anafranil, and Prozac.

The FDA's sudden ban on L-tryptophan seemed justified at first, at least if all you heard about it was in the popular media: an epidemic of a severely debilitating and sometimes fatal disease known as eosinophilia–myalgia syndrome (EMS) was found to infect frequent users of L-tryptophan. In the name of protecting the consumer, this certainly appeared to be sufficient grounds for taking it off the shelves. But subsequently it was discovered that the EMS sufferers were limited to only those people who had used L-tryptophan manufactured by a particular company (Showa Denko/Japan), in a particular batch. Furthermore, the specific EMS contaminant in this batch was isolated by the Centers for Disease Control, proving conclusively that the culprit was a bad batch, not the supplement itself. Nonetheless, the FDA's consignment of L-tryptophan to the status of "Investigational Unapproved New Drug" remains in effect to this day. You cannot buy it legally anywhere in this country.

At the time of L-tryptophan's untimely demise, it accounted for something on the order of $180 million in sales, none of which found its way into the coffers of the major drug manufacturers. Yet in the meantime, the FDA has approved Anafranil, Ciba-Geigy's prescription drug for serotonin enhancement, to be used by depressives and obsessive-compulsives. Anafranil's listed possible side effects in the *Physicians' Desk Reference* include seizures (frequent), psychosis, elevated liver enzymes, and a high rate of sexual dysfunction (particularly in males), all apparently acceptable risks by FDA standards. Anafranil costs about a buck and a half a hit.

Likewise, Eli Lilly's antidepressant, Prozac, another serotonin enhancer, recently passed $1 billion in annual sales. In addition to having the same possible side effects as Anafranil, Prozac has been implicated as the precipitant in some suicides and violent assaults.

But perhaps the most interesting comparison is with the Upjohn sleeping pill, Halcion. The great majority of L-tryptophan's users bought the supplement to combat insomnia, and they were able to get a good night's sleep for roughly one-fifth of the cost of Halcion (not to mention the cost of a trip to the doctor to get a prescription for it). But the larger curiousness is the fact that Halcion has been reported to cause depression and induce suicide in enough cases to warrant taking it off the market in Great Britain and Sweden. No problem for the FDA, however.

Let me be perfectly clear: any conspiracy theory worth its salt needs to have evidence of collusion, and I have not come across any such evidence linking the FDA's unwarranted ban of L-tryptophan to the manufacturers of its more expensive prescription competitors.

But it sure does give a fellow pause.

First Find a Cure, Then Design a Disease

Let's say that the FDA in good faith decides to review the professor-businessman's petition to classify melatonin as a prescription drug. What are the issues the agency has to consider? First, it has to determine that melatonin actually cures a disease, inhibits the development of a disease, or alleviates the symptoms of one. If it does none of the above, it is not a drug, only an innocuous supplement, one that its manufacturers can make no claims for.

Note that the over-the-counter bottle of melatonin on your drugstore or health-food-store counter does not say on its label, CURES INSOMNIA. By law, only a drug can claim to cure a bona fide disease like insomnia. The health writer Michael Castleman has pointed out that a grocer could find himself in deep legal doodoo if he were to post a sign over his garlic bin saying, GARLIC REDUCES CHOLESTEROL. This, even though the *Annals of Internal Medicine* and several other medical journals have published research definitively demonstrating that eating garlic reduces cholesterol. By contrast, the prescription drug cholestyramine (Questran), which costs over a buck a day (about forty times the cost of a few cloves of garlic), can tout its cholesterol-reducing properties all it wants.

Are we starting to see a pattern here?

The next question the FDA has to address when considering the professor-businessman's petition is whether melatonin is safe, including whether its side effects are acceptable, you know, like it only runs the risk of causing seizures, psychoses, elevated liver enzymes, or violent outbursts.

Here is where the whole mechanism by which the FDA decides whether a drug becomes an affordable over-the-counter product or a restricted and prohibitively expensive prescription drug clearly works against the consumer's best interests. The burden of testing a drug for safety and efficacy is on the producer of the drug. Therefore no company will go to the formidable expense of thoroughly testing a product unless it can be guaranteed sole propriety of that product and a hefty profit on it once they prove it to be safe and effective. On average, it takes a new drug twelve years, 100,000 pages of paperwork, and $100–$400 million to obtain FDA approval (although with pressure from AIDS victims, this process has been sped up in recent years).

Obviously, no pharmaceutical company is going to spend this kind of time and money on, say, garlic, which would appear to be unpatentable and is relatively cheap to produce—there is literally no percentage in it. Or, as James Duke, Ph.D., a senior botanist at the U.S. Department of Agriculture, put it, "Who in their right mind would spend $1 million on a new drug application for garlic?"

So what options does this leave the entrepreneurial professor?

For one, he can produce evidence which proves that unless melatonin is taken under an M.D. or D.O.'s supervision (hence, by prescription), the melatonin-taker runs a substantial risk of running into telephone poles. Knowing what I do about the relative harmlessness of melatonin when taken in low doses, the professor would be hard-pressed to convince me of this risk.

Yet there is another tack that the professor-businessman could take and this, I believe, is the most insidious of them all: He could design a disease for which melatonin is the cure! Is this beginning to sound like Alice in Wonderland? Well, hold on to your rabbit, because FDA policy has a pronounced Lewis Carroll quality when it comes to determining exactly what constitutes a disease. The FDA operates under a dictum that says, in effect: "If it ain't a disease, you can't cure it; therefore if it ain't a disease, you can't prescribe a drug for it."

That only seems logical, right?

But with this dictum in mind, pharmaceutical companies go to great trouble and expense to get those conditions for which they have chemical cures deemed diseases.

For example, one relatively new "mental disease" that was recently codified in psychiatry's bible of legitimate diseases, the *Diagnostic Statistical Manual of Mental Disorders* (DSM-4), is attention deficit hyperactivity disorder (ADHD). This happened after Ciba-Geigy Pharmaceuticals had discovered that Ritalin, an amphetamine compound which they had long produced for weight loss, had the paradoxical effect in intractable children of making them better-behaved and more attentive students. But, of course, it could not be prescribed for these children unless their condition was officially a disease, so Ciba-Geigy got busy lobbying the editors of the DSM and the governors of the FDA to make it so. They brought in teachers and educational psychologists to claim that habitual fidgetiness constituted a learning disorder. They brought in brain anatomists to demonstrate (rather lamely, most neurologists believe) that children who do not focus well on their studies, and who cannot sit still for long periods, have a different cerebral structure from normal students. Ciba's success at this enterprise can be seen in the estimated two million American ADHD children who take Ritalin daily, and in the millions of dollars in annual sales that Ciba garners from their cure.

But is ADHD really a mental disease or only a social problem? And if only the latter, should doctors be prescribing drugs for it? I only raise these questions here to suggest the arbitrariness in assigning the label "disease" to some conditions and not to others, and to posit the idea that corporate profit and FDA politics may sometimes be involved in making these decisions. In any event, we are all left in murky waters: What mental and physical conditions should we call diseases? And at what stage of those conditions should we intercede with medicines?

The Ultimate Disease: Old Age

As I write, there is a new disease for which a cure already exists on the drawing boards: age-associated memory impairment (AAMI).

If drug companies are successful in making this disease official, the payoff will be monumental. At last count, American pharmaceutical companies were developing over 140 mind- and memory-enhancing drugs in their laboratories, ready for when the AAMI floodgates open. But if and when they do open, it will be both good and bad news for the consumer.

The good news is that "Young Brain Drugs" will at last be able to be legally prescribed by physicians. And once legitimized, these drugs may be prescribed for any patient a doctor decides can benefit from them, regardless of his age. The bad news, of course, is that prescription drugs are by their very nature expensive, among other reasons because the cost of testing them is passed on to the consumer. Furthermore, knowledgeable consumers in their thirties, forties, and fifties will have to hunt around for doctors who share their conviction that the time to combat age-associated memory impairment is before it becomes a problem—not after.

Undoubtedly, most doctors and FDA professionals will argue against prophylactic use of Young Brain Drugs by young and middle-aged men and women. They will insist on seeing testable symptoms of the disease before prescribing a drug for it. This is because they know something they don't really want you to think about, namely that Young Brain Drugs may not merely prevent diseases like senility and Alzheimer's, they may actually enhance the powers of undiseased minds. (By the same token, Ritalin unsurprisingly makes "undiseased" students even more attentive in the classroom.) Young Brain Drugs have the potential to make all of us, regardless of age, smarter, more alert, and more capable than we would normally be without them.

But for the FDA, simply enhancing our mental or physical capabilities with a drug goes against its inveterate Puritanism. The flip side of the You-Need-A-Disease-If-You've-Got-A-Cure protocol is that any drug that can simply make us better than we would be normally is off-limits. This attitude seems to trickle down from the prohibition against performance-enhancing drugs in competitive sports; these drugs strike most of us as constituting an unfair advantage. But does the analogy to brain performance-enhancing drugs hold? Is it an unfair advantage to become smarter and have a better memory by taking a drug? Advantage over whom? And what if such a drug were available to everyone—who's got the advantage then?

In any event, the practical question remains: What are testable symptoms of age-associated memory impairment and where do the doctors draw the line? When someone forgets the words to "The Star-Spangled Banner"? When she regularly forgets where she parked her car? When he frequently walks upstairs to get something and then forgets what it is he wanted?

These are murky waters.

The renowned advocate of preventative medicine, Dr. William Regelson has proposed an eminently sensible formula for cutting through this morass. He asserts that aging itself should be considered a life-threatening disease. And that the time to start curing it is right now.

End of problem. Bravo, Dr. Regelson!

Before I Forget

Here is what worries me personally: I have had much more pharmacological training than the average physician. However, suppose I felt that, in the last few years, I had a discernable drop in my ability to read and memorize research papers. And that I went to my neurologist to be sure there was nothing serious going on, and she ruled out the presence of any type of clinically recognizable cognitive problem. And that she told me "You simply have the normal small amount of short-term memory loss and ability to concentrate that many of us get as we reach our forties."

So, suppose I then researched the scientific literature on, say, Piracetam, the smart drug marketed under many different names in Europe where it is prescribed for senile dementia, alcoholism, vertigo, dyslexia, and even Alzheimer's disease. And in this literature, I discovered that Piracetam had also been shown to enhance the cognitive abilities of many people who have no clinical disorders, which would hardly surprise me. Thus, I would have the possibility of using a pharmaceutical compound for something other than for treatment of a recognized disease.

Now, let us say that after scrutinizing the literature, I concluded that this drug was extremely safe in both the short and long term, so I saw no reason for not giving it a try. I could order some of this compound from various sources in Europe; however, the FDA, through Customs, could confiscate my package containing Piracetam when it arrived in this country. What the FDA would essentially be saying to me is: This drug is not approved for use in any known disease here, and we will decide what you can and cannot use, because you are incapable of making these decisions yourself.

Of course, I know that what this usually means is that a U.S. pharmaceutical company either has a patent on a similar drug or is working on one, and that I would only be able to buy that drug with a physician's prescription when it was approved.

One option I would have, of course, is I could go to one of my colleagues who is a physician and he could write me a prescription for Piracetam; then it would be perfectly all right in the eyes of the FDA for me to import and use this drug, despite the fact that the physician might know absolutely nothing about this compound.

Although the FDA approves drugs for particular diseases, it does not limit the way a physician uses an approved drug—she can prescribe it for absolutely any disorder for which she believes it will be useful. Furthermore, a physician also has the right to prescribe drugs from overseas that have no approved use in the United States.

But the hypocrisy of this arrangement is obvious: it's okay in the FDA's eyes for a physician to prescribe an approved or unapproved drug for use in any medical condition, even if this doctor has no idea what the therapeutic result will be. However, someone without benefit of a medical-school degree who has done his homework on these drugs cannot on his own cognizance choose to try a pharmaceutical compound for cognitive enhancement. This is true even if that compound has been approved for use in other countries and has well-documented safety record. But most distressing, this is true even if published results show that the drug or compound does indeed enhance cognitive functions, or act as a potent antioxidant, or is in any other way effective at extending your Youthspan.

A Brief Moment of Paranoia

Indulge me for just one moment here and let me ask an impertinent and quite possibly paranoid question: Who would stand to lose substantial profits if a large portion of the population were able to inexpensively expand its Youthspan?

First, geriatric physicians would face a huge drop in business. So would their colleagues in cardiology, oncology, and pulmonary diseases, not to mention a good number of social workers and nurses. Then, of course, institutions like nursing homes and "mature housing" (one of the fastest growing markets in the U.S.) would find their profits leveling off even as the aging population was growing. And the big loser, of course, would be the pharmaceutical industry—extended years of good health translates directly into contracted drug revenues.

But I promised no conspiracy theories, right? Surely no self-respecting health-care organization could possibly sabotage any product or practice that would improve the general population's health and extend their Youthspan just to maximize its profits, could it?

I certainly hope not.

But in the meantime, I intend to do everything within my power to ensure that everyone has the necessary knowledge and opportunities to live young for a very long time.

Resources

Finding an Anti-Aging Physician

One of the most important aspects of getting on board the "Youthspan train" is to find a physician who is knowledgeable about the huge amount of information that is now in the published scientific literature. This covers the use of various types of behavior modifications, dietary changes, herbs, antioxidants, smart drugs, synthetic drugs, etc., that are involved in preventing disease and prolonging the Youthspan. There are only two types of physicians in the United States who are fully licensed to practice medicine, the M.D.s, and the D.O.s (D.O.s are doctors of osteopathy, who go through essentially the same training that M.D.s do, but are generally more inclined to use nondrug or nonsurgical intervention for a problem, if at all possible).

It is not an easy task to find such a physician, as currently only a small percentage of physicians are even interested in preventative medicine, much less educated about it. As I have mentioned elsewhere in this book, the vast majority of most M.D.'s and D.O.'s time and training is spent focusing on the recognition and diagnosis of existing disease, and applying known treatments (mostly drugs and surgery) to that disease. As I have also said, the unfortunate part about this approach is that, although it works very well for acute disease and trauma, it is mostly either ineffective, or effective for only a short period of time, for age-related, chronic degenerative disease, which has no cure. Therefore, the logical approach is to prevent, or greatly delay the onset of, chronic age-related disease, and that's what this book is all about.

It is very difficult to simply list physicians who describe themselves as practicing preventative medicine. That's because it is impossible for me, or anyone else for that matter, to completely check the background of every single one of those physicians who claim to practice preventative medicine, and say with certainty that they do indeed have extensive training in the new and emerging field of anti-aging and preventative medicine.

However, there are at least a few good places to start to seek such a physician. One is to call the American Academy of Anti-Aging Medicine (A4M). This academy, of which I am a member, was founded in 1992 by Dr. Ronald Klatz and Dr. Robert Goldman. It currently has 4,000 members from forty countries and is growing quite rapidly. The headquarters of the A4M is located in Chicago, Illinois. Many, if not most, of these A4M members are licensed M.D.s and D.O.s who are interested in practicing antiaging medicine, with most of the remainder being Ph.D. scientists who do research in the area of antiaging medicine.

In December 1997, the American Board of Antiaging Medicine, which was formed by A4M, offered the first certification examination to M.D.s and D.O.s signifying specialty expertise in the new discipline of antiaging medicine and therapeutics. To become certified in antiaging medicine, the candidate must, in addition to being a fully licensed M.D. or D.O., demonstrate at least five years in clinical practice, pass both written and oral examinations, and pass the scrutiny of the examining board for academic, professional, and ethical standards. The person must also have at least 200 hours of continuing medical education in a related field of medicine, such as preventative cardiology, sports medicine, nutrition, endocrinology, or the pharmacology of aging, among others.

This certification examination will ultimately lead to subspecialty recognition and status as a qualified practitioner in the new clinical practice of antiaging medicine. The good news is that the A4M now produces a yearbook of participating physicians, with information about their location, as well as the antiaging therapies and protocols they offer. You can call, write, or fax the A4M to inquire about getting one of these yearbooks. It costs $12.95 for non-members of the A4M, plus $4.95 shipping and handling. This is certainly a prime source to use in your search to find an antiaging physician who may live near you. The following is all the information you will need:

The American Academy of Anti-Aging Medicine
1341 W. Fullerton, Suite 111
Chicago, IL 60614
Internet address: http://www.worldhealth.net/
Phone: (773) 528–4333
Fax: (773) 528–5390

Furthermore, I would like to note that the A4M is not some "quack" organization. This is the nation's largest society of physicians and scientists finally coming together to prevent the diseases of aging, as opposed to treating these diseases after they occur.

In fact, the A4M has finally gotten the FDA to see the light. In a groundbreaking, unexpected move in February 1997, the FDA (led by Dr. Jack Longmire, an FDA clinical investigator in Rockville, Maryland) has asked the A4M to help it in the development of a totally new class of drugs, to be called "antiaging therapeutics." This was hailed by the president of the A4M, Dr. Ronald Klatz, as a major breakthrough in the struggle to change the way that physicians look at disease. You can follow the progress of these negotiations on the Internet, either through updates at the A4M website (listed above), or at the FDA's Internet site (simply do a search, and use "FDA" as the searchword, and you will get their Web address).

Another good way to find a competent physician in your area who is knowledgeable about antiaging medicine, and who is willing to help you in your efforts to extend your Youthspan, is to call your state Medical Licensure Board to see if there is a division of alternative, or more appropriately, "complementary" medicine (since most of this type of medicine "complements" traditional medicine). Some states, including Maine, the state I work in, have these listings, and they may be able to steer you to a competent physician who can help you in your efforts to learn about true disease prevention.

Finally, another way to find such a physician is to simply ask around, starting with your own physician. Ask her if she would be willing to help you in your endeavors to live disease-free for a long period of time, and if so, whether she actually knows anything about the practice of antiaging medicine. If it is a busy clinic with people being shuffled in and out in fifteen minutes, you can be almost certain that nobody there is trained in, or involved with antiaging medicine.

Of course, your physician may very well know other physicians in the area who might be able to help you, and may provide you with names. Remember, you don't necessarily have to leave your current physician, whom you may have a good relationship with. In fact, your regular physician may be the most appropriate avenue for you if you get seriously ill. I'm simply saying that if your physician knows nothing about antiaging and true preventative medicine (other than the "catch-it-in-the-early-stages" protocols, like PAP smears, breast and prostate exams, etc., which are not really preventative in nature), then you might want to retain the services of a prevention-oriented physician, whose job it will be to keep you out of the office of your regular physician.

Naturopaths

Another type of healthcare professional who may actually be more useful to you than most M.D.s and D.O.s when it comes to true preventative medicine are the naturopathic doctors (N.D.s). N.D.s go through a four-year medical curriculum, but do not do a residency in a specialized area like M.D.s and D.O.s. In addition, they cannot perform major surgery, and are limited in the medical tests they can order, as well as the drugs they can prescribe.

You will find most N.D.s in a general, private practice, although some may concentrate on specific modalities, such as pediatrics, gynecology, allergies, etc. If you want to know more about what N.D.s do, how they are trained, and how to contact one in your area, visit the "Naturopathic Medicine Network" on the Internet, at http://www.pandamedicine.com/index.html. Or, if you simply wish to find out if N.D.s are licensed to practice in your state, look in your Yellow Pages and call your state's Medical Licensure Board, as each state is different regarding what types of health-care professionals they allow to practice there.

Again, to summarize, a very useful rule of thumb here is that using a physician trained in antiaging medicine as your advocate in your endeavor to maximize your Youthspan is an excellent idea. You need to use common sense, however. If you are already sick with some particular type of disease, you should seek the help of a conventional physician, assuming the disease you have is readily treatable by conventional medicine. If, however, you are already sick with a disease that is not well treated or curable with conventional medicine, then seeking alternative treatments through alternative medicine is also a good idea.

Smart Drug Information

For those of you interested in purchasing any of the so-called smart drugs that I described, your best bet is from the sources listed below.

With specific regards to smart drugs, and more information about them, call, write, or visit the website of the Cognitive Enhancement Research Institute (CERI) in California. Their addresses are:

CERI
P.O. Box 4029
Menlo Park, CA 94026
Phone: (415) 321–2374
Website: http://www.ceri.com/

The CERI website is an excellent source of information regarding smart drugs and other life-enhancing products, including a frequently updated listing of physicians that can be used to supervise and monitor your use of smart drugs. It also includes information on how to obtain overseas or in Mexico smart drugs such as Piracetam that are currently not available in the U.S., and what the FDA's policy is on the personal importation of such compounds. I list various sources here for those people without Internet access.

To purchase the software I described in Chapter 6 for measuring objective changes in response to smart drugs, write to:

Cognitive Diagnostics
12 Corporate Plaza, Suite 150
Newport Beach, CA 92660
Fax: (714) 718-1112
Website: http//www.brain.com

International Sources
Discovery of Mexico

c/o B&B Freight Forwarding
5025 N. Central Avenue, Suite 619
Phoenix, AZ 85012

Call toll free: 888–687–0884 for ordering or pricing changes. (For ordering outside of the U.S. see International Antiaging Systems below.)

Drugstore O.L. Skouvara & Co.

Epaminonda 82, Thiva 32200, Greece
Fax-011–30–1–883–1680

This company has access to over 7,000 different pharmaceuticals. When requesting price quote, please provide generic chemical name whenever possible. This company was formerly known as Vipharm.

World Health Services

P.O. Box 20, CH-2822
Courroux, Switzerland

World Health Services provides numerous smart drugs and other FDA-unapproved European pharmaceuticals.

International Merchandise Procurement

P.O. Box 336,
Phuket 83000, Thailand
Fax: 011–66–76–38–1057

A source for smart drugs and longevity medicines.

Biorica Internacional, S.A.

S.A. P.O. Box 5263 FR-RD,
8911 Rifferswil, Switzerland
Phone: 011–41–61–422–1292, Fax: 011–41–61–422–1289

Complete supplement service including smart drugs, hormone-replacement therapy, vitamins, minerals and health-food store items. Orders taken by fax. The company takes American Express and

VISA. Prescription service available for items sold by Biorica. Ask for its complete catalog of products.

Masters Marketing Company, Ltd.

Masters House—No. 1, Marlborough Hill
Harrow Middlesex HA1 1TW, England
Phone: 011–44–181–424–9400, Fax: 011–44–181–427–1994

This company provides European pharmaceuticals, and it now accepts VISA and MasterCard credit cards. The above phone number is dedicated to U.S. customers.

Big Ben Export Co. (Tudor Trading Co.)

P.O. Box 146, Mill Hill
London NW7 3DL, England

This company exports (and imports) pharmaceuticals.

International Antiaging Systems

IAS, P.O. Box 337
Guernsey, Channel Islands, Great Britain
Phone: 011–44–541–514144
Fax: 011–44–541–514145 or 011–44–7000–IASLTD (427583)

IAS specializes in antiaging therapies. It sells most of the popular smart drugs including L-tryptophan and GHB. The company now carries Discovery-brand liquid L-deprenyl. VISA and MasterCard accepted except to the European Union.
E-mail address: iasltd@attmail.com

Victoria Apotheke

Bahnhofstrasse 71, Postfach
CH–8021 Zurich, Switzerland
Phone: 011–41–1–211–24–32, Fax: 011–41–1–221–23–22

Victoria Pharmacy is a mail-order source that is well known in AIDS-activist circles. It is known for locating hard-to-find pharmaceuticals, and has been very helpful to many contending with life-threatening disease. Victoria also carries a wide range of smart drugs and life-extension items. For more information you can call or fax it at the above numbers. Its website address is: www.access.ch/victoria_pharmacy; Compuserve address is 101372, 1667; Internet: victoriaapotheke@access.ch

Quality Health, Inc.
401 Langham House
29–30 Margaret Street
London W1N 7LB, England
Fax: 011–44–171–580–2043

Quality Health, Inc. is offering very competitive prices. It offers the most popular smart drugs as well as L-trytophan and acetyl-L-carnitine, and accepts payment by personal check, international money order, VISA, and MasterCard. Normal delivery time is twenty-one days but the company will post orders by express mail for an additional fee. Information voicemail for U.S. and Canadian customers: 1–800–350–7270.
Website: www.qhi.co.uk
E-mail: sales@qhi.co.uk

Vitality Health Products
23/1 Caro Mio, Sark, Guernsey GY9 OSE
Channel Islands, Great Britain
Phone: 011–44–1481–832–617, Fax: 011–44–1481–832–515

Vitality Health Products supplies a broad selection of smart drugs, as well as other popular pharmaceutical products. Inquiries are invited. All products are branded and sourced mainly in Thailand. The firm states, "Delivery approximately 21 days from receipt of order," and accepts VISA, MasterCard, and American Express.
Internet: 106123.3540@compuserve.com

Era-Bond Laboratories
72 New Bond Street
London W1Y 9DD, England
Fax: 011–44–171–499–3417

Era-Bond carries GHB, and other popular smart and prosexual drugs such as bromocriptine, deprenyl, dexfenfluramine, DHEA, L-dopa, Hydergine, melatonin, Piracetam, tryptophan, etc. Payments can be made by money order or official check.

NutroPharm
Bredaweg 45, 1324 XT Almere, The Netherlands
Phone: 011–31–20–682–7870, Fax: 011–31–20–681–5947

NutroPharm is of special interest to European buyers, as it carries many products originating in the United States. These include a wide range of food supplements such as smart nutrients, energy products, Durk Pearson & Sandy Shaw's designer foods, multisupplements, weight-loss products, fitness products, prosexual nutrients, phytonutrients, etc. Payment policy: Payment in advance with (Euro) check, international money order, or bank transfer.

Domestic Supplement Sources

The following are supplement sources in the U.S. for such things as antioxidants, vitamins, minerals, herbs, amino acids, and some hormones (a selection of the smart drugs, such as phosphatidylserine and Gingko biloba, can also be bought domestically). You should call them and check prices, as some may be slightly less expensive than others at any given time. Keep in mind that currently there is no regulation of these companies for quality control of their products (i.e., a guarantee that what is in them is what they say is in them). However, many of these companies do quality-control checks, and make them available. My advice is to ask them for copies of quality-control reports for any herbs, amino acids, fatty acids, or hormones you may be purchasing (vitamins and minerals are usually not a problem). I have not heard of any actions against any of the companies I have listed here for any reasons.

Smart Basics
1626 Union Street
San Francisco, CA 94123
Toll-free: (800) 878–6520

Smart Basics carries an extensive line of Pearson & Shaw nutrient-based products; request its free catalog and newsletter. The company carries both DHEA and pregnenolone. It takes VISA, MasterCard, American Express, and Discover credit cards. Fax: (415) 351–1348. Website: www.smartbasic.com; E-mail: smartnet@sirius.com

LifeLink
750 Farroll Road
Grover Beach, CA 93433
Toll-free: (888) 433–5266 Fax: (805) 473–2803 Local: (805) 473–1389.

LifeLink sells DHEA (liquid and capsules), pregnenolone, 5-hydroxy-tryptophan, and colloidal silver.

Due to issues related to use patents, LifeLink has stopped selling NADH. Court hearings are pending. It now takes VISA and MasterCard. Website: www.lifelinknet.com.

Olympia
1765 Garnet #66
San Diego, CA 92109
Phone: (619) 275–6477 Fax: (619) 276–2831

Olympia is a discount source for brain products like DMAE, acetyl-L-carnitine, phosphatidylserine, MegaMind, NADH, DHEA, and hard-to-find products. Olympia is the U.S. representative for International Antiaging Systems.
E-mail: olympia@smart-drugs.com; Website: www.smart-drugs.com

Life Services Supplements
3535 Route 66
Neptune, NJ 07753
Toll-free: (800) 542–3230 Local: (908) 922–0009
Fax: (908) 922–LFAX

LSS carries the complete line of Pearson & Shaw designer foods and personal-care products. It also publishes a monthly newsletter.

Peggy's Health Center
151 First Street
Los Altos, CA 94022
Toll-free: (800) 862–9191 Local: (415) 948–9191

Peggy's carries many easy- and hard-to-find nutrient/supplement products including progesterone cream and NADH. Peggy's will ship throughout the world.

The Vitamin Shop
Toll-free: (800) 223–1216

The shop carries 1,000 mg PCA (pyroglutamate) tablets.

L&H Vitamins
37–10 Crescent Street
Long Island City, NY 11101
Toll-free: (800) 221–1152 Fax: (718) 361–1437

A large mail-order supplier with an extensive catalog.

Ecological Formulas
1061-B Sharly Circle
Concord, CA 94518
Toll-free: (800) 888–4585 Fax: (510) 827–2636

This firm carries Cardiovascular Research-brand melatonin capsules.

Vitamin Express
1428 Irving Street
San Francisco, CA 94122
Phone: (415) 564–8160 Fax: (415) 564–3156

1400 Shattuck Avenue
Berkeley, CA 94709
Phone: (510) 841–1798

45 Camino Alto
Mill Valley, CA 94901
Phone: (415) 389–9671

Vitamin Express is a full-spectrum supplement store with over 5,000 products, at discount prices. It carries DHEA, pregnenolone, DMAE, acetyl-L-tyrosine, phosphatidylserine, N-acetyl carnitine, beta-1, 3-glucans, alpha lipoic acid, and other smart and specialty nutrients from many companies. Vitamin Express handles mail orders throughout the world and is glad to handle customer supplement inquiries. It also publishes a newsletter, and has a website at: www.vitaminexpress.com

Nutrition Plus

4747 E. Elliot Road, Suite 29
Phoenix, AZ 85044
Toll-free: (800) 241–9236 Fax: (303) 872–3862

Nutrition Plus carries a wide range of supplement products with a specialty in smart-nutrient supplements.

KAL Supplements

6415 De Soto Avenue
Woodland Hills, CA 91365
Toll-free: (800) 755–4525

KAL is a distributor to health-food stores. If it can't direct you to a local store, it will fill your order directly.

Vitamin Research Products

3579 Highway 50 East
Carson City, NV 89701
Toll-free: (800) VRP-24HR

VRP carries a complete line of dietary supplements including 3 mg and 750 mcg melatonin capsules. The company mail-orders worldwide.

Pharmacognosy-22
Suite 5288, 1945 East Ridge Road
Rochester, NY 14622
Toll-free: (800) 56-NEURON (563–8766)

This company supplies a broad spectrum of amino acids in powder form, and also carries selected vitamins, nutrients, proteins, and cognitive-enhancement products.

NutriGuard Research
P. O. Box 865
Encinitas, CA 92023
Toll-free: (800) 433–2402 Local: (619) 942–3223

NutriGuard carries arginine pyroglutamate, phosphatidylcholine, Staminex, glucosamine, and numerous other multinutrient formulas.

ASTAK
29949 S.R. 54 West
Wesley Chapel, FL 33543
Phone: (813) 973–7902

ASTAK distributes the liquid DHEA product developed by Discovery Experimental & Development, Inc.

BIOS Biochemicals
8987–309 E. Tanque Verde, Suite #340
Tucson, AZ 85749
Phone: (520) 326–7610 Fax: (520) 362–2385

BIOS sells powdered amino acids (including L-tryptophan) for veterinary and pet-food use in quantities from 50 grams to multiple kilos. Its tryptophan is USP (pharmaceutical) grade, greater than 99.5 percent purity, and is "free of pyrogen and EBT." BIOS also carries DHEA and pregnenolone. Call or write for a price list. Request a price list by E-mail: rsturtz@primenet.com. BIOS now takes credit cards.

Life Enhancement Products, Inc.

P. O. Box 751390
Petaluma, CA 94955
Toll-free: (800) 543–3873 Fax: (707) 769–8016 Local: (707) 762–6144

Life Enhancement Products is a source for supplements, including sublingual melatonin and high-purity DHEA. It also has a line of supplements formulated by Ward Dean, M.D., and Durk Pearson & Sandy Shaw. LEP accepts credit cards and ships within twenty-four hours. Its newsletter (Life Enhancement News) is available by request.

River of Life Natural Foods

6220 Lower York Road
New Hope, PA 18938
Local phone: (215) 862–5134

River of Life Natural Foods stocks numerous smart nutrients that may be of interest, including an extensive assortment of Source Naturals' products. Ask for free catalog.

Tierra Marketing International (TMI)

223 N. Guadalupe, Suite 285
Santa Fe, NM 87501
Toll-free: (800) 736–6253 Fax: (505) 982–0698

TMI is a worldwide source for original-formula, procaine-based Gerovital (GH#3). It also carries 5-hydroxy-L-tryptophan, NADH, pregnenolone, and DHEA. VISA, MasterCard, and American Express accepted. Contact Tierra for prices, as well as details of its 1994 court victory defending GH#3 against the FDA.
E-mail: VitaMan@rt66.com Website: www.rt66.com/vitaman/

Beyond a Century

HC 76, Box 200
Greenville, ME 04441
Toll-free: (800) 777–1324 Fax: (207) 695–2492

Performance nutritional products. Amino acid mixtures, antioxidant formulas, athletic and weight-loss formulas, meal replacements, sterol creams, skin and hair products, etc. Hundreds of products. E-mail: beyacent@aol.com.

Douglas Laboratories
600 Boyce Road
Pittsburgh, PA 15205
Toll-free: 888-DOUGLAB

GTC Nutrition Company
Box 843
Broomfield, CO 80038
Toll-free: (800) 522–4682

Natrol
20731 Marilla Street
Chatsworth, CA 91311
Toll-free: (888) 262–8765

Nature's Way Products
10 Mountain Springs Parkway
Springville, UT 84663
Phone: (801) 489–1520

Twin Laboratories
Ronkonkoma, NY 11779
Phone: (516) 467–3140

Tyson Labs
Wakunga of America Co.
23501 Madero
Mission Viejo, CA 92691
Toll-free: (800) 421–2998

Another good source of domestic nutritional products are the General Nutrition Centers, which are a national chain of stores selling health supplements, and can be found in most malls across the U.S. Just check your Yellow Pages.

Diagnostic Testing Sites

The following sites offer various diagnostic tests that can be very useful to you and your physician in evaluating your current health, and preventing early onset of future health problems.

Genox Corporation
1414 Key Highway
Baltimore, MD 21230
Phone: (410) 347–7616 Fax: (410) 347–7617

Genox offers several diagnositic tests to aid you, or you and your physician, in your overall health-maintenance plan. Genox has tests for all the major antioxidants regularly found in blood, and has also developed several "oxidative stress profile" tests, which estimate your body's capacity to deal with the free radicals that play such an important role in aging and disease. Genox also offers advice on what the tests mean, and how to approach rectifying any problems which might show up on tests. Call Genox or visit its Website for more specific information. E-mail: genox@aol.com; Website: http://www.genox.com

Doctors Data Laboratories Inc.
P.O. Box 111
170 W. Roosevelt Road
West Chicago, IL 60185
Toll-free: (800) 323–2784 Fax: (708) 231–9190

Doctors Data has been around for about twenty-five years, helping doctors and patients most specifically in the area of elemental analysis of hair, whole blood, packed blood cells, and urine, as well as comprehensive amino acid analysis of blood and urine samples. These types of tests can provide useful information about the body status with regards to important, as well as toxic, minerals. Write or call the company, and it will send you a packet with more specific information regarding the tests it does, insurance coverage of the tests, and the value of these tests to your long-term health.

Great Smokies Diagnostic Laboratory
63 Zillicoa Street
Asheville, NC 28801–1074
Toll-free: (800) 522–4762 Fax: (704) 253–1127

The Great Smokies Diagnostic Lab (GSDL) is also involved in many types of preventative health testing. Some of the services the GSDL offers are oxidative stress profiles, osteoporosis risk evaluation, and parasitology tests. It also offers a detoxification profile, which is essentially a series of tests that evaluates your body's, capacity to handle various toxins. GSDL will also do an intestinal permeability test, as a "leaky gut" has been shown to be clinically correlated with a number of disorders, including chronic inflammatory diseases. Write or call GSDL for a packet that describes these tests, the costs and potential benefits of these tests, and how to work with your doctor to have these tests performed. E-mail: cs@gsdl.com. Website: http://www.gsdl.com

Vitamin Research Products
3579 Highway 50 East
Carson City, NV 89701
Toll-free: (800) 877–2447 Fax: (800) 877–3292

Vitamin Research Products (VRP) was mentioned in the section on domestic-supplement sources, because it manufactures many types of nutrient supplements. Now VRP offers hormone-testing kits, which allow you to measure levels of certain hormones in the comfort of your home, without drawing blood. These kits involve the use of saliva to estimate plasma levels of various hormones (the salivary levels are correlated to the blood levels), and come with instructions on how to collect the samples. The samples will then be sent off to a diagnostic lab and hormone levels will be measured, and the results, along with an interpretation, will be mailed to you. These tests do not require a physician's prescription, but you should certainly get a knowledgeable physician's input on interpreting the results, if you do not understand them. There are kits available for at least seven hormones at this time, including DHEA, melatonin, testosterone, progesterone, total progestins, estradiol, and total estrogens. E-mail: vrp@delphi.com

Health-Related Websites

I have selected the following websites as good places to visit to get excellent, updated medical information on current health problems, a healthy lifestyle, avoidance of disease, and general medical information.

The National Women's Health Information Center
Provides links to federal information organizations, as well as resources from hundreds of private organizations. To find out about women's health issues, access a news-clipping service, and research abstracts on a broad range of topics, visit the Internet site at http://www.4woman.org/

Alternative Medicine Homepage
An excellent site to visit on the Internet is the Alternative Medicine Homepage. The web address is http://www.pitt.edu/~cbw/altm.html. This website can give you lots of information about links to other similar websites, mailing lists, and newsgroups regarding alternative medicine and health.

Office of Alternative Medicine
Believe it or not, the National Institutes of Health actually has an Office of Alternative Medicine (OAM), which was established in 1992. The Congressional mandate establishing the OAM stated that the purpose was to "facilitate the evaluation of alternative medical treatment modalities" for the purpose of determining their effectiveness, and to help integrate treatments into mainstream medical practice. The OAM does not serve as a referral agency for various alternative-medicine treatment modalities or individual practitioners. However, you can contact the OAM and ask for one of its "information packets," which will provide you with information on such things as what is alternative medicine, and where your tax dollars are being spent regarding different types of research on alternative-medicine therapies. The address for the OAM is:

OAM Information Center
Office of Alternative Medicine, NIH
9000 Rockville Pike, Room 5B-38
Bethesda, MD 20892
Telephone: (301) 402–2466 Fax: (301) 402–4741
Website: http://www.pitt.edu/~cbw/oam.html

UT-Houston Center for Alternative-Medicine Research

One of the better websites I have found regarding nontraditional medicine research is the University of Texas (UT)-Houston Center for Alternative-Medicine Research. This center is dedicated to investigating the effectiveness of alternative medicines used specifically for cancer prevention and control. The University of Texas Center for Alternative Medicine (UT-CAM) is in fact one of ten alternative medicine research centers established by the NIH's OAM (described above) to evaluate alternative therapies. This center is cofunded by the National Cancer Institute. The University of Texas Center is the only OAM-supported institution focused solely on alternative and complementary treatments for cancer. The website for UT-CAM is: http://www.sph.uth.tmc.edu/www/utsph/utcam/index.htm

Of course, the UT-CAM is just one research center funded by the NIH's OAM, and it is only involved with cancer treatment and prevention. To find out about other research sites in the U.S. that are carrying out OAM-funded research in alternative methods in the treatment or prevention of such things as pain, addiction, allergy, asthma, stroke, and HIV, call the NIH Alternative Medicine Hotline at: (888) 644–6226.

Physicians' Guide to the Internet

Filled with lots of the latest medical information on existing disease, as well as some promising preventative strategies. Although this website is predominantly for physicians, if you are knowledgeable in healthcare, you will find it very interesting.
Web address: http://www.webcom.com/pgi/welcome.html

Medscape

Another website that is primarily geared to physicians, but contains many late-breaking stories regarding all types of disease, and prevention as well. Also provides free access to Medline, a computer program which allows you to search for publications in the medical literature. Web site: http://www.medscape.com/

Doctors' Guide to the Internet
As the name implies, another website primarily for doctors, but full of great medical information, and updated regularly. Website: http://www.pslgroup.com/docguide.htm

Medicine Links
A very useful website that can link you up to almost any medical topic you would like to know about, and then some. One of my favorite "hook-up" sites. Website: http://www.hooked.net/users/wcd/listmed.htm

National Institute on Aging
The National Institute on Aging (NIA) is one of the National Institutes of Health, the principal biomedical research agency of the United States government. The NIA promotes healthy aging by conducting and supporting biomedical, social, and behavioral research and public education. You can access its homepage on the Internet.
Website: http://www.nih.gov/nia/
The Public Information Office at the National Institute on Aging produces science-based educational materials on a wide range of topics related to health and aging. Subjects cover specific diseases and health conditions, treatments, and research. The materials are for use by the general public, patients and family members, health professionals, voluntary and community organizations, and the media. For single copies, send request by E-mail to: niainfo@access. digex.net, or call toll-free: (800) 222–2225, (800) 222–4225 (TTY) between 8:30 A.M. and 5:00 P.M., eastern standard time.

Food and Nutrition Information Center
The Food and Nutrition Information Center (FNIC) is one of several information centers at the National Agricultural Library (NAL), Agricultural Research Service (ARS), United States Department of Agriculture (USDA). Website: http://www.nalusda.gov/fnic/
The FNIC homepage is a great place to start your Internet search

for nutrition information. They have many publications on nutrition and also provide an excellent jumping-off point for other good sources of nutrition information.

Diagnostic Procedures

Are you concerned about having a medical test, and don't feel that the reasons for doing it, or the benefits and risks, have been explained to you adequately? Try going to the following website and looking up your test: http://www.healthgate.com/HealthGate/free/dph/static/a.index.shtml#authors

Diagnostic Procedures, with Key Word Index, details 294 common and less common procedures, and is offered as a handy comprehensive, yet concise, quick reference for practitioners and other healthcare professionals, but also for knowledgeable patients. The authors, as practicing physicians, have attempted to provide up-to-date information with emphasis on consensus interpretations and practical considerations concerning the diagnostic procedures described in their specialty section. Be sure to discuss with your doctor any new questions you may have concerning your test before you make any decision about whether to have a test done or not.

Pub Med

Pub Med is a medical database opened to the public in June of 1997. It was developed by the National Center for Biotechnology Information, and contains all sorts of health information from more than 3,800 publications. It can be found at: ncbi.nlm.nih.gov/pubmed/

Tufts Nutrition Navigator

The Tufts University Nutrition Navigator (TUNN) is the first on-line rating and review guide that solves the two major problems Web users have when seeking nutrition information: how to quickly find information best suited to their needs and whether to trust the information they find. The TUNN is designed to help you sort through the large volume of nutrition information on the Internet and find accurate, useful information you can trust.

Website address: http://www.navigator.tufts.edu

Bibliography

Chapter One: The Biology of Aging

Ames, B.N., Shigenaga, M.K., and T.M. Hagen. 1993. "Oxidants, Antioxidants, and the Degenerative Diseases of Aging." *Proceedings of the National Academy of Sciences* (U.S.A.). 90:7915.

Ando, S., Kon, K., Aino, K., and Y. Totani. 1990. "Increased Levels of Lipid Peroxides in Aged Rat Brain as Revealed by Direct Assay of Peroxide Values." *Neuroscience Letters.* 113:199.

Bredesen, D.E. 1996. "Keeping Neurons Alive: The Molecular Control of Apoptosis (part I)." *The Neuroscientist.* 2(3):181–190.

Carney, J.M., Starke-Reed, P.E., Oliver, C.N., Landum, R.W., Cheng, M.S., Wu, J.F., and R.A. Floyd. 1991. "Reversal of Age-Related Increase in Brain Protein Oxidation, Decrease in Enzyme Activity, and Loss in Temporal and Spatial Memory by Chronic Administration of the Spin-Trapping Compound N-Tert-butyl-a-phenylnitrone." *Proceedings of the National Academy of Sciences* (U.S.A.). 88:3633.

Chen, Q., Fischer, A., Reagan, D.J., Yan, L.J., and B.N. Ames. 1995. "Oxidative DNA Damage and Senescence of Human Diploid Fibroblast Cells." *Proceedings of the National Academy of Sciences* (U.S.A.). 92:4337.

Cutler, R.G. 1984. "Antioxidants, Aging, and Longevity." In: *Free Radicals and Biology.* W.A. Pryor, ed. pp. 371–428. Academic Press, New York.

Forster, M.J., Dubey, A., Dawson, K.M., Stutts, W.A., Lal, H., and R.S. Sohal. 1996. "Age-Related Losses of Cognitive Function and Motor Skills in Mice Are Associated with Oxidative Protein Damage in the Brain." *Proceedings of the National Academy of Sciences* (U.S.A.). 93:4765–4769.

Greider, C.W. 1991. "Telomorase Is Processive." *Molecular and Cellular Biology.* 11(9):4572–4580.

Gutteridge, J. 1993. "Free Radicals in Disease Processes: a Compilation of Cause and Consequence." *Free Radical Research Communications.* 19:141.

Harley, C.B., Futcher, A.B., and C.W. Greider. 1990. "Telomeres Shorten During Aging of Human Fibroblasts." *Nature.* 345(6274):458–460.

Harman, D. 1956. "Aging: A Theory Based on Free Radical and Radiation Chemistry." *Journal of Gerontology*. 11:298–300.

Harman, D. 1992. "Free Radical Theory of Aging." *Mutation Research*. 275:257.

Hayflick, L. 1965. "The Limited In Vitro Lifetime of Human Diploid Cell Strains." *Experimental Cell Research*. 37:614–636.

Lebovitz, R., Zhang, H., et al. 1996. "Neurodegeneration, Myocardial Injury, and Perinatal Death in Mitochondrial Superoxide Dismutase-Deficient Mice." *Proceedings of the National Academy of Sciences* (U.S.A.). 93:9782.

Mann, D.M., Yates, P.O., and J.E. Stamp. 1978. "The Relationship Between Lipofuscin Pigment and Ageing in the Human Nervous System." *Journal of the Neurological Sciences*. 37:83–93.

Miquel, J. 1991. "An Integrated Theory of Aging as a Result of Mitochondrial DNA Mutation in Differentiated Cells." *Archives of Gerontology and Geriatrics*. 12:99.

Nandy, K. 1985. "Lipofuscin as a Marker of Impaired Homeostasis in Aging Organisms." In: *Homeostatic Function and Aging*. B. Davis and W. Wood, eds. Raven Press, New York.

Orr, W.C., and R.S. Sohal. 1994. "Extension of Lifespan by Overexpression of Superoxide Dismutase and Catalase in Drosophila Melanogaster." *Science*. 263:1128.

Park. J.W., Choi, C.H., et al. 1996. "Oxidative Status in Senescence-Accelerated Mice." *Journal of Gerontology*. 51A(5):B337.

Raff, M., Barres, B., et al. 1993. "Programmed Cell Death and the Control of Cell Survival: Lessons from the Nervous System." *Science*. 262:695.

Short, R., Williams, D., and D. Bowden. 1997. "Circulating Antioxidants as Determinants of the Rate of Biological Aging in Pigtailed Macaques *Macaca nemestrina*)." *Journal of Gerontology*. 52A(1):B26.

Chapter Two: The Free-Radical Hit List

The Immune System

Chandra, R.K. 1989. "Nutritional Regulation of Immunity and Risk of Infection in Old Age." *Immunology*. 67:141.

Ershler, W.B. 1993. "The Influence of Aging and Immune System on Cancer Incidence and Progression." *Journal of Gerontology*. 48:B3.

Harbige, L. 1996. "Nutrition and Immunity, with Emphasis on Infection and Autoimmune Disease." *Nutrition and Health*. Vol. 10. pp. 285–312.

Meydani, S., Meydani, M., et al. 1997. "Vitamin E Supplementation and In Vivo Immune Response in Healthy Elderly Subjects." *Journal of the American Medical Association*. 277(17):1380.

Santos, M., Meydani, S., et al. 1996. "Natural Killer Cell Activity in Elderly Men is enhanced by Beta Carotene Supplementation." *American Journal of Clinical Nutrition*. 64:772.

Cancer

Comstock, G., et al. 1991. "Prediagnostic Serum Levels of Carotenoids and Vitamin E as Related to Subsequent Cancer in Washington County, Maryland." *American Journal of Clinical Nutrition*. 53:2605.

Comstock, G., et al. 1992. "Serum Retinol, Beta Carotene, Vitamin E, and Selenium as Related to Subsequent Cancer of Specific Sites." *American Journal of Epidemiology*. 135:115.

Gey, K. 1993. "Propects for the Prevention of Free Radical Disease, Regarding Cancer and Cardiovascular Disease." *British Medical Bulletin*. 49(3):679.

Helzlsouer, K. J., Block, G., Blumberg, J., et al. 1994. "Summary of the Round-Table Discussion on Strategies for Cancer Prevention: Diet, Food, Additives, Supplements, and Drugs. *Cancer Research.* (suppl.) 54:2044S–2051S.

Lewis, C. E. 1988. "Disease Prevention and Health Promotion Practices of Primary Care Physicians in the United States." *American Journal of Preventative Medicine.* 4 (suppl.):9–16.

Nomura, A., Stemmermann, G., et al. 1985. "Serum Vitamin Levels and the Risk of Cancer of Specific Sites in Men of Japanese Ancestry in Hawaii." *Cancer Research.* 45:2369.

Richter, C., Park, J.W., and B.N. Ames. 1988. "Normal Oxidative Damage to Mitochondrial and Nuclear DNA is Extensive." *Proceedings of the National Academy of Sciences* (U.S.A.). 85:6465.

Vogelstein, B. And K. W. Kinsler. 1993. "The Multistep Nature of Cancer." *Trends in Genetics.* 9:138–141.

Cataracts

Hankinson, S., Willett, W., et al. 1992. "A Prospective Study of Cigarette Smoking and Risk of Cataract Surgery in Women." *Journal of the American Medical Association.* 268(8):994.

Jaques, P., and L. Chylack Jr. 1991. "Epidemiologic Evidence of a Role for the Antioxidant Vitamins and Carotenoids in Cataract Prevention." *American Journal of Clinical Nutrition.* 53:352S.

Knekt, P., Heliovaara, M., et al. 1992. "Serum Antioxidant Vitamins and Risk of Cataract." *British Medical Journal.* 305:1392.

Leskie, M., Chylack, L., and S.Y. Wu. 1991. "The Lens Opacities Case-Control Study." *Archives of Opthalmology.* 109:244.

Varma, S. 1991. "Scientific Basis for Medical Therapy of Cataracts by Antioxidants." *American Journal of Clinical Nutrition.* 53:335S.

Cardiovascular Disease

Gaziano, J., Manson, J., et al. 1992. "Dietary Antioxidants and Cardiovascular Disease." *Biochimica et Biophysica Acta.* 669:249.

Gey, K. 1989. "Plasma Vitamins E and A Inversely Related to Mortality from Ischemic Heart Disease in Cross-Cultural Epidemiology." *Annals of the New York Academy of Sciences.* 570:268.

Gey, K. 1990. "The Antioxidant Hypothesis of Cardiovascular Disease: Epidemiology and Mechanisms." *Biochemical Society Transactions.* 18:1041.

Gey, K. 1992. "Vitamin E and Other Essential Antioxidants Regarding Coronary Heart Disease: Risk Assessment Studies. A review." In: *Vitamin E: Biochemistry and Clinical Applications.* L. Packer and J. Fuchs, eds. pp. 589–633. M. Dekker, New York.

McGinnis. J.M., and W.H. Foege. 1993. "Actual Cause of Death in the United States." *Journal of the American Medical Association.* 270(18):2207.

Salonen, J., Salonen, R., et al. 1988. "Relationship of Serum Selenium and Antioxidants to Plasma Lipoproteins, Platelet Aggregability, and Prevalent Ischemic Heart Disease in Eastern Finnish Men." *Atherosclerosis.* 70:155.

Brain Aging

Ando, S., Kon, K., Aino, K., and Y. Totani. 1990. "Increased Levels of Lipid Peroxides in Aged Rat Brain as Revealed by Direct Assay of Peroxide Values." *Neuroscience Letters.* 113:199.

Corral-Debrinski, M., Horton, T., Lott, M.T., Shoffner, J.M., et al. 1992. "Mitochondrial DNA Deletions in Human Brain: Regional Variability and Increase with Advanced Age." *Nature Genetics.* 2:324.

Cortopassi, G. A., Shibata, D., Soong, N. W., and N. A. Arnheim. 1992. "A Pattern of Accumulation of a Somatic Deletion of Mitochondrial DNA in Aging Human Tissues." *Proceedings of the National Academy of Sciences* (U.S.A.). 89:7370–7374.

Gotz, M.E., Freyberger, A., and P. Reiderer. 1990. "Oxidative stress: a Role in the Pathogenesis of Parkinson's Disease." *Journal of Neural Transmission.* (suppl.). 29:241.

Jenner, P. 1991. "Oxidative Stress as a Cause of Parkinson's Disease." *Acta Neurologica Scandinavica.* (suppl.). 136:6.

Matsuo, M., Gomi, F. and M. M. Dooley. 1992. "Age-Related Alterations in Antioxidant Capacity and Lipid Peroxidation in Brain, Liver and Lung Homogenates of Normal and Vitamin E-Deficient Rats." *Mechanisms of Ageing and Development.* 64:273–292.

Merocci, P., McGarvey, U., Kaufman, A.E., Koontz, D., et al. 1993. "Oxidative Damage to Mitochondrial DNA Shows Marked Age-Dependant Increases in Human Brain." *Annals of Neurology.* 34:609.

Poon, L.W. 1985. "Differences in Human Memory with Aging: Nature, Causes, and Clinical Implications." In: *Handbook of the Psychology of Aging.* J.E. Birren and K.W. Schaie, eds. pp. 427–462. Van Nostrand Reinhold, New York.

Scarpa, M., Rigo, A., Viglino, P., Stevanato, R., Bracco, F., and L. Battistin. 1987. "Age Dependence of the Level of the Enzymes Involved in the Protection Against Active Oxygen Species in the Rat Brain." *Proceedings of the Society for Experimental Biology and Medicine.* 185:129–133.

Smith, M., Sayre, L., et al. 1995. "Radical AGEing in Alzhemier's Disease." *Trends in Neurosciences.* 18(4):173.

Volicer, L. and P. B. Crino. 1990. "Involvement of Free Radicals in Dementia of the Alzheimer Types: a Hypothesis." *Neurobiology of Aging.* 11:567–571.

Zs.-Nagy, I. 1991. "Dietary Antioxidants and Brain Aging: Hopes and Facts." In: *The Potential for Nutritional Modulation of the Aging Process.* D. Ingram, G. Baker, and N. Shock, eds. Food and Nutritional Press Inc., Trumbull, Connecticut.

Chapter Three: No Brainer

Baskys, A., Reynolds, J., and P. Carlen. 1990. "NMDA Depolarizations and Long-Term Potentiation are Reduced in the Aged Rat Neocortex." *Brain Research.* 530:142.

Black, J., Isaacs, K., et al. 1990. "Learning Causes Synaptogenesis, whereas Motor Activity Causes Angiogenesis in Cerebellar Cortex of Adult Rats." *Proceedings of the National Academy of Sciences* (U.S.A.). 87:5568.

Bliss, T., and G. Collingridge. 1993. "A Synaptic Model of Memory: Long-Term Potentiation in the Hippocampus." *Nature.* 361:31.

Castorina, M., Ambrosini, A., et al. 1994. "Age-Dependant Loss of NMDA Receptors in Hippocampus, Striatum, and Frontal Cortex in the Rat: Prevention by Acetyl-L-Carnitine." *Neurochemical Research.* 19(7):795.

Greenough, W., Withers, G., and C. Wallace. 1990. "Morphological Changes in the Nervous System Arising from Experience: What is the Evidence They are Involved in Learning and Memory?" In: *The Biology of Memory.* L. Squire and E. Lindenlaub, eds. Schattauer Verlag, Stuttgart.

Snowdon, D., Kemper, S. et al. 1996. "Linguistic Ability in Early Life and Cognitive

Function and Alzheimer's Disease Late in Life." *Journal of the American Medical Association.* 275(7):528.

Stern, Y., Gurland, B., et al. 1994. "Influence of Education and Occupation on the Incidence of Alzheimer's Disease." *Journal of the American Medical Association.* 271(13):1004.

Stoll, S., Hartman, H., Cohen, S.A., and W.E. Muller. 1993. "The Potent Free Radical Scavenger Alpha Lipoic Acid Improves Memory in Aged Mice: Putative Relationship to NMDA Receptor Deficits." *Pharmacology Biochemistry and Behavior.* 46:799.

Tamaru, M., Yoneda, Y., et al. 1991. "Age-Related Decreases in the NMDA Receptor Complex in the Rat Cerebral Cortex and Hippocampus." *Brain Research.* 542:83.

Vernadakis, A. 1996. "Glia-Neuron Intercommunications and Synaptic Plasticity." *Progress in Neurobiology.* 49:185.

Zhang, M., Katzman, R., et al. 1990. "The Prevalence of Dementia and Alzheimer's Disease in Shanghai, China: Impact of Age, Gender, and Education." *Annals of Neurology.* 27(4):428.

Chapter Four: The Young Brain/Young Mind/Young Body Cycle

Arbel, I., Kadar, T., Sibermann, M., and A. Levy. 1994. "The Effect of Long-Term Cortisol Administration on Hippocampal Morphology and Cognitive Performance of Middle-Aged Rats." *Brain Research.* 657:227.

Ben-Eliyahu, S., Yirmiya, R., et al. 1991. "Stress Increases Metastatic Spread of a Mammary Tumor in Rats: Evidence for Mediation by the Immune System." *Brain Behavior and Immunity.* 5:193.

Bergsma, J. 1994. "Illness, the Mind, and the Body: Cancer and Immunology, an Introduction." *Theoretical Medicine.* 15:337.

Dachar, S., Kadar, T., Robinson, B., and A. Levy. 1993. "Cognitive Deficits Induced in Young Rats by Long-Term Cortisol Administration." *Behavioral and Neural Biology.* 60:103.

Dale, D.C., and R.G. Petersdorf. 1973. "Corticosteroids and Infectious Diseases." *Medical Clinics of North America.* 57:1277.

Goya, L., Rivero, F., and A. Pascual-Leone. 1995. "Glucocorticoids, Stress, and Aging." In: *Hormones and Aging.* P. Timiras, ed. CRC Press, Boca Raton, Florida.

Gruber, B., 1988. "Immune System and Psychological Changes in Metastatic Cancer Patients Using Relaxation and Guided Imagery: a Pilot Study." *Scandinavian Journal of Behavioral Therapy.* 17:25.

Harbuz, M., and S. Lightman. 1992. "Stress and the Hypothalamo-Pituitary-Adrenal Axis: Acute, Chronic, and Immunological Activation." *Journal of Endocrinology.* 134:327.

Kerr, D., Campbell, L., Applegate, M., Brodish, A., and P.W. Landfield. 1991. "Chronic Stress-Induced Acceleration of Electrophysiological and Morphometric Biomarkers of Hippocampal Aging." *Journal of Neuroscience.* 11:1316.

Lupien, S., Gaudreau, B., et al. 1997. "Stress-Induced Declarative Memory Impairment in Healthy Elderly Subjects: Relationship to Cortisol Reactivity." *Journal of Clinical Endocrinology and Metabolism.* 82(7):2070.

Maddin, K., and S. Livnat. 1991. "Catecholamine Action and Immunologic Reactivity." In: *Psychoneuroimmunology.* 2nd edition. R. Ader, N. Cohen, and D. Felten, eds. pp. 283–310, Academic Press, New York.

Maier, S., Watkins, L., and M. Fleshner. 1994. "Psychoneuroimmunology. Interface

Between Behavior, Brain, and Immunity." *American Psychologist*. December 1994.

Rinehart, J., Sagone, A., Balcerzak, S., Ackerman, G., and A. LaBuglio. 1975. "Effects of Corticosteroid Therapy on Human Monocyte Function." *New England Journal of Medicine*. 292:236.

Sapolsky, R. M. 1985. "A Mechanism for Glucocorticoid Toxicity in the Hippocampus: Increased Neuronal Vulnerability to Metabolic Insults." *Journal of Neuroscience*. 5:1227.

Sapolsky, R.M., Krey, L., and B.S. McEwen. 1985. "Prolonged Glucocorticoid Exposure Reduces Hippocampal Neuron Number: Implications for Aging." *Journal of Neuroscience*. 5:1222.

Sapolsky, R.M. 1996. "Why Stress Is Bad for Your Brain." *Science*. 273:749.

Schaffner, A., and T. Schaffner. 1987. "Glucocorticoid-Induced Impairment of Macrophage Antimicrobial Activity: Mechanisms and Dependance on the State of Activation." *Reviews of Infectious Diseases*. 9:S620.

Schleifer, S., Keller, S., et al. 1983. "Suppression of Lymphocyte Stimulation Following Bereavement." *Journal of the American Medical Association*. 250:374.

Schlesinger, M., and Y. Yodfat. 1996. "Psychoneuroimmunology, Stress, and Disease." In: *Psychoneuroimmunology, Stress, and Infection*. H. Friedman, T. Klein, and A. Friedman, eds. pp. 127–136, CRC Press. Boca Raton, Florida.

Selye, H. 1936. "A Syndrome Produced by Diverse Noxious Agents." *Nature*. 38:32.

Speigel, D., et al. 1989. "Effect of Psychosocial Treatment on Survival of Patients with Metastatic Breast Cancer." *Lancet*. 2:888.

Chapter Six: Smart Tools 1: Smart Drugs and Nutrients

Gingko Biloba

Eckmann, F. 1990. "Cerebral Insufficiency: Treatment with Gingko Biloba Extract. Time of Onset of Effect in a Double-Blind Study with 60 Inpatients." *Fortschritte der Medizin*. 108(29):557.

Grassel, E. 1992. "Effect of Gingko Biloba Extract on Mental Performance. Double-blind Study Using Computerized Measurement Conditions in Patients with Cerebral Insufficiency." *Fortschritte der Medizin*. 110(5):73.

Hindmarch, I. 1986. "Activity of Gingko Biloba Extract on Short-Term Memory." *Presse Medicale*. 15(31):1592.

Hofferberth, B. 1989. "The Effect of Gingko Biloba Extract on Neurophysiological and Psychometric Measurement Results in Patients with Psychotic Organic Brain Syndrome. A Double-Blind Study against Placebo." *Arzneimittelforschung*. 39(8):918.

Le Bars, P., et al. 1997. "A Placebo-Controlled Double-Blind Randomized Trial of an Extract of Gingko Biloba for Dementia." *Journal of the American Medical Association*. 278(16):1327.

Meyer, B. 1986. "Multicenter Randomized Double-Blind Drug versus Placebo Study of the Treatment of Tinnitus with Gingko Biloba Extract." *Presse Medicale*. 15(31):1562.

Rai, G., Shovlin, C., and K. Wesnes. 1991. "A Double-Blind, Placebo-Controlled Study of Gingko Biloba Extract (Tanakan) in Elderly Outpatients with Mild to Moderate Memory Impairment." *Current Medical Research and Opinion*. 12(6):350.

Sikora, R., et al. 1989. "Gingko Biloba Extract in the Therapy of Erectile Dysfunction." *Journal of Urology*. 141:188A.

Subhan, Z., and I. Hindmarch. 1984. "The Psychopharmacological Effects of Gingko

Biloba Extract in Normal Healthy Volunteers." *International Journal of Clinical Pharmacology Research.* 4(2):89.

Taillandier, J., Ammar, A., et al. 1986. "Treatment of Cerebral Aging Disorders with Gingko Biloba Extract. A Longitudinal Multicenter Double-Blind Drug versus Placebo Study." *Presse Medicale.* 15(31):1583.

Acetyl-L-Carnitine

Bowman, B. 1992. "Acetyl-L-Carnitine and Alzheimer's Disease." *Nutrition Review* (U.S.A.) 50(5):142.

Castorina, M., Ambrosini, A., et al. 1994. "Age-Dependant Loss of NMDA Receptors in Hippocrampus, Striatum, and Frontal Cortex in the Rat: Prevention by Acetyl-L-Carnitine." *Neurochemical Research.* 19(7):795.

Cippoli, C., and G. Chiari. 1990. "Effects of Acetyl-L-Carnitine on Mental Deterioration in the Aged: Initial Results." *Clinica Terapeutica* (Roma). 6(suppl.):479.

Lino, A., et al., 1992. "Psychofunctional Changes in Attention and Learning under the Action of Acetyl-L-Carnitine in 17 Young Subjects. A Pilot Study of its Use in Mental Deterioration." *Clinica Terapeutica* (Roma). 140(6):569.

Sinforiani, E., Iannuccelli, M., et al. 1990. "Neuropsychological Changes in Demented Patients Treated with Acetyl-L-Carnitine." *International Journal of Clinical Pharmacology Research.* 10(1–2):69.

Tempesta, E., Troncon, R., et al. 1990. "Role of Acetyl-L-Carnitine in the Treatment of Cognitive Deficit in Chronic Alcoholism." *International Journal of Clinical Pharmacology Research.* 10(1–2):101.

Hydergine

Bertoni-Freddari, C., Giuli, C., Pieri, et al. 1987. "The Effect of Chronic Hydergine Treatment on the Plasticity of Synaptic Junctions in the Dentate Gyrus of Aged Rats." *Journal of Gerontology.* 42(5):482.

Emmenegger, H., and W. Meier-Ruge. 1968. "The Actions of Hydergine on the Brain." *Pharmacology.* 1:65.

Hollister, L.E. 1988. "Ergoid Mesylates and the Treatment of Senile Dementias." In: *Perspectives in Psychopharmacology: A Collection of Papers in Honor of Earl Usdin.* Alan R. Liss, New York.

Schneider, L.S., and J.T. Olin. 1994. "Overview of Clinical Trials of Hydergine in Dementia." *Archives of Neurology.* 51(8):787.

Steurer, G, Fitscha, P., et al. 1989. "Effects of Hydergine on Platelet Deposition on "Active" Human Carotid Artery Lesions and Platelet Function." *Thrombosis Research.* 55(5):577.

Phosphatidylserine

Crook, T.H. et al. 1991. "Effects of Phosphatidylserine on Age-Associated Memory Impairment." *Neurology.* 41:644.

Maggioni, M., Picotti, G., et al. 1990. "Effects of Phosphatidylserine Therapy in Geriatric Patients with Depressive Disorders." *Acta Psychiatrica Scandinavica.* 81(3):265.

Palmeiri, G., et al. 1987. "Double-Blind Controlled Trial of Phosphatidylserine in Subjects with Senile Mental Deterioration." *Clinical Trials Journal* (Amsterdam). 24:73.

Rabboni, M., Maggioni, F., et al. 1990. "Neuroendocrine and Behavioral Effects of Phosphatidylserine in Elderly Patients with Abiotrophic or Vascular Dementia, and Mild Depression. A Preliminary Trial." *Clinical Trials Journal* (United Kingdom). 27(3):230.

Rosadini, G. et al. 1991 "Phosphatidylserine: Quantitative EEG Effects in Healthy Volunteers." *Neuropsychobiology.* 24:42.

Piracetam and Derivatives

Chaudry, H. Najam, N., et al. 1992. "Clinical Use of Piracetam in Epileptic Patients." *Current Therapeutical Research, Clinical and Experimental.* 52(3):355.

Fiorvavanti, M., et al. 1991. "A Multi-Center, Double-Blind Controlled Study of Piracetam versus Placebo in Geriatric Patients with Non-Vascular Mild to Moderate Impairment in Cognition." *New Trends in Clinical Neuropharmacology.* 5(1):27.

Friedman, E., Sherman, K., et al. 1981. "Clinical Response to Choline plus Piracetam in Senile Dementia: Relation to Red-Cell Choline Levels." *New England Journal of Medicine.* 304(24):1490.

Itil, T., Menon, G., et al. 1986. "CNS Pharmacology and Clinical Therapeutic Effects of Oxiracetam." *Clinical Neuropharmacology.* 9(suppl. 3):S70.

Lenegre, A., et al. 1988. "Specificity of Piracetam's Anti-Amnesic Activity in Three Models of Amnesia in the Mouse." *Pharmacology Biochemistry and Behavior.* 29:625.

Maina, G., Fiori, L., et al. 1989. "Oxiracetam in the Treatment of Primary Degenerative and Multi-Infarct Dementia: A Double-Blind Placebo-Controlled Study." *Neuropsychobiology.* 21(3):141.

Mindus, P. Cronholm, B., et al. 1976. "Piracetam: Induced Improvement in Mental Performance. A Controlled Study on Normally Aging Individuals." *Acta Psychiatrica Scandinavica.* 54:150.

Pilch, H., and W. Muller. 1988. "Piracetam Elevates Muscarinic Cholinergic Receptor Density in the Frontal Cortex of Aged Mice but Not of Young Mice." *Psychopharmacology.* 94:74.

Schaffler, K., and W. Klausnitzer. 1988. "Randomized, Placebo-Controlled, Double-Blind Cross-Over Study of Antihypoxidotic Effects of Piracetam Using Psychophysiological Measures in Healthy Volunteers." *Arzneimittelforschung.* 38(2):288.

Centrophenoxine (Lucidril)

Marcer, D., and S. Hopkins. 1977. "The Differential Effects of Meclofenoxate on Memory Loss in the Elderly." *Age and Ageing.* 6:123.

Nagy, I., and R. Floyd. 1984. "Electron Spin Resonance Spectroscopic Demonstration of the Hydroxyl Free Radical Scavenger Properties of DMAE in Spin-Trapping Experiments Confirming the Molecular Basis for the Biological Effects of Centrophenoxine." *Archives of Gerontology and Geriatrics.* 3(4):297.

Pek, G., and T. Fulop. 1989. "Gerontopsychological Studies Using NAI ('Nürnberger Alters-Inventar') on Patients with Organic Psychosyndrome (DSM III, Category 1) Treated With Centrophenoxine in a Double Blind, Comparative, Randomized Clinical Trial." *Archives of Gerontology and Geriatrics.* 9(1):17.

Riga, S., and D. Riga. 1974. "Effects of Centrophenoxine on the Lipofuscin Pigments in the Nervous System of Old Rats." *Brain Research.* 72:265.

Semsei, I. 1985. "Superoxide Radical Scavenging Ability of Centrophenoxine and its Salt Dependence In Vitro." *Journal of Free Radicals in Biology and Medicine.* 1(5–6):403.

Sharma, D., Maurya, A.K., and R. Singh. 1993. "Age-related Decline in Multiple Unit Action Potentials of CA3 Region of Rat Hippocampus: Correlation with Lipid Peroxidation and Lipofuscin Concentration and the Effect of Centrophenoxine." *Neurobiology of Aging.* 14(4):319.

Sharma, D., and R. Singh. 1995. "Centrophenoxine Activates Acetylcholinesterase

Activity in Hippocampus of Aged Rats." *Indian Journal of Experimental Biology.* 33(5):365.

Stancheva, S., and L. Alova. 1988. "Effect of Centrophenoxine, Piracetam and Aniracetam on the Monoamine Oxidase Activity in Different Brain Structures of Rats." *Farmakol Toksikol.* 51(3):16.

Chapter Eight: Basic Mega-Chicken Soup Tools I: Supplements

Beta Carotene and the Carotenoids

Alpha Tocopherol, Beta Carotene Cancer Prevention Study Group (ATBC Trial). 1994. "The Effect of Vitamin E and Beta Carotene on the Incidence of Lung Cancer and Other Cancers in Male Smokers." *New England Journal of Medicine.* 330(15):1029.

Blot, W., Li, J. Y., et al. 1993. Nutrition Intervention Trials in Linxian, China: Supplementation with Specific Vitamin/Mineral Combinations, Cancer Incidence, and Disease-Specific Mortality in the General Population ("General Population Trial"). *Journal of the National Cancer Insitute.* Issue of September 15.

Di Mascio, P., Murphy, M., and H. Sies. 1991. "Antioxidant Defense Systems: the Role of Carotenoids, Tocopherols, and Triols." *American Journal of Clinical Nutrition.* 53:194S.

Foote, C.S., and R.W. Denny. 1968. "Chemistry of Singlet Oxygen, VII. Quenching by Beta Carotene." *Journal of the American Chemical Society.* 90:6233.

Hughes, D., Wright, A., et al. 1997. "The Effect of Beta Carotene Supplementation on the Immune Function of Blood Monocytes From Healthy Male Non-Smokers." *Journal of Laboratory and Clinical Medicine.* 129(3):309.

Kramer, T., and B. Burri. 1997. "Modulated Mitogenic Proliferative Responsiveness of Lymphocytes in Whole Blood Cultures After a Low Carotene Diet and Mixed-Carotenoid Supplementation in Women." *American Journal of Clinical Nutrition.* 65:871.

Lepage, G., Champagne, J., Ronco, N., Lamarre, A., et al. 1996. "Supplementation with Carotenoids Corrects Increased Lipid Peroxidation in Children with Cystic Fibrosis." *American Journal of Clinical Nutrition.* 64:87.

Li, J.Y., Taylor, P., et al. 1993. Nutrition Intervention Trials in Linxian, China: Multiple Vitamin/Mineral Supplementation, Cancer Incidence, and Disease-Specfic Mortality among Adults with Esophageal Dysplasia ("Dysplasia Trial"). *Journal of the National Cancer Institute.* Issue of September 15.

Niki, E., Noguchi, N., Tsuchihashi, H., and N. Gotoh. 1995. "Interaction Among Vitamin C, Vitamin E, and Beta Carotene." *American Journal of Clinical Nutrition.* 62(suppl.):1322S.

Omenn, G., Goodman, G., et al. 1996. "Effects of a Combination of Beta Carotene and Vitamin A on Lung Cancer and Cardiovascular disease ('CARET Trial')." *New England Journal of Medicine.* 334:1150.

Phillips, R., Kikendall, J., et al. 1993. "Beta Carotene Inhibits Rectal Mucosal Ornithine Decarboxylase Activity in Colon Cancer Patients." *Cancer Research.* 53:3723.

Santos, M., Meydani, S., et al. 1996. "Natural Killer Cell Activity in Elderly Men is Enhanced by Beta Carotene Supplementation." *American Journal of Clinical Nutrition.* 64:772.

Stich, H., Mathew, B., et al. 1991. "Remission of Precancerous Lesions in the Oral Cavity of Tobacco Chewers and Maintenance of the Protective Effect of Beta Carotene and Vitamin A." *American Journal of Clinical Nutrition.* 53:298S.

Watson, R., et al. 1991. "Effect of Beta Carotene on Lymphocyte Subpopulations in Elderly Humans: Evidence for a Dose-Response Relationship." *American Journal of Clinical Nutrition*. 53:90.

Yeum, K.J., Booth, S., et al. 1996. "Human Plasma Carotenoid Response to the Ingestion of Controlled Diets High in Fruits and Vegetables." *American Journal of Clinical Nutrition*. 64:594.

Ziegler, R., Subar, A., et al. 1992. "Does Beta Carotene Explain Why Reduced Cancer Risk is Associated with Vegetable and Fruit Intake?" *Cancer Research* (suppl.). 52:2060S.

Vitamin E and the Tocopherols

Behl, C., Davis, J., et al. 1992. "Vitamin E Protects Nerve Cells from Amyloid Beta Protein Toxicity." *Biochemical and Biophysical Research Communications*. 186(2):944.

Dieber-Rotheneder, M., Puhl, H., et al. 1991. "Effect of Oral Supplementation with D-Alpha Tocopherol on the Vitamin E Content of Human Low-Density Lipoproteins and Resistance to Oxidation." *Journal of Lipid Research*. 32:1325.

Di Mascio, P., Murphy, M., and H. Sies. 1991. "Antioxidant Defense Systems: the Role of Carotenoids, Tocopherols, and Triols." *American Journal of Clinical Nutrition*. 53:194S.

Kushi et al., 1996. "Dietary Antioxidant Vitamins and Death From Coronary Heart Disease in Post-Menopausal Women." *New England Journal of Medicine*. 334:1156.

Meydani, S., Meydani, M., et al. 1997. "Vitamin E Supplementation and In Vivo Immune Response in Healthy Elderly Subjects." *Journal of the American Medical Association*. 277(17):1380.

Monji, A., Nobumitsu, M., et al. 1994. "Effect of Dietary Vitamin E on Lipofuscin Accumulation with Age in the Rat Brain." *Brain Research*. 634:62.

Poulin, J., Cover, C., et al. 1996. "Vitamin E Prevents Oxidative Modification of Brain and Lymphocyte Band 3 Proteins During Aging." *Proceedings of the National Academy of Sciences* (U.S.A.). 93:5600.

Regnstrom, J., Nilsson, J., et al. 1996. "Inverse Relation between Concentration of Low-Density Lipoprotein Vitamin E and Severity of Coronary Artery Disease." *American Journal of Clinical Nutrition*. 63:377.

Rimm, E., Stampfer, M., et al. 1993. "Vitamin E Consumption and the Risk of Coronary Heart Disease in Men." *New England Journal of Medicine*. 328(20):1450.

Sano, M., Ernesto, C., et al. 1997. "A Controlled Trial of Selegiline, Alpha Tocopherol, or Both as Treatment for Alzheimer's Disease." *New England Journal of Medicine*. 336(17):1216.

Stampfer, M. and E. Rimm. 1995. "Epidemiological Evidence for Vitamin E in Prevention of Cardiovascular Disease." *American Journal of Clinical Nutrition*. 62(suppl.):1365S.

Steiner, M., Glantz, M., and A. Lekos. 1995. "Vitamin E plus Aspirin Compared with Aspirin Alone in Patients with Transient Ischemic Attacks." *American Journal of Clinical Nutrition*. 62(suppl.):1381S.

Vitamin C

Cook, J., and E. Monsen. 1977. "Vitamin C, the Common Cold, and Iron Absorption in Man." *American Journal of Clinical Nutrition*. 30:235.

Frei, B., England, L., and B.N. Ames. 1989. "Ascorbate Is an Outstanding Antioxidant in Human Blood Plasma." *Proceedings of the National Academy of Sciences* (U.S.A.). 86:6377.

Levine, M. Dhariwal, K., et al. 1995. "Determination of Optimal Vitamin C Requirements in Humans." *American Journal of Clinical Nutrition.* 62(suppl.):1347S.

Levine, M., et al. 1996. "Vitamin C Pharmacokinetics in Healthy Volunteers: Evidence for a Recommended Dietary Allowance." *Proceedings of the National Academy of Sciences* (U.S.A.). 93:3704.

Stocker, R., and B. Frei. 1991. "Endogenous Antioxidant Defense in Human Blood Plasma." In: *Oxidative Stress: Oxidants and Antioxidants.* H. Sies, ed. pp, 213–243, Academic Press, New York.

Wayner, D.D., Burton, G.W., Ingold, K., Barclay, L., et al. 1987. "The Relative Contribution of Vitamin E, Urate, Ascorbate, and Proteins To the Total Peroxyl Radical-Trapping Antioxidant Activity of Human Blood Plasma." *Biochimica et Biophysica Acta.* 924:408.

Glutathione

Bernard, G. 1991. "N-Acetyl-Cysteine in Experimental and Clinical Acute Lung Injury." *American Journal of Medicine.* 91:54.

Forman, H., Liu, R.M., and M. Ming Shi. 1995. "Glutathione Synthesis in Oxidative Stress." In: *Biothiols in Health and Disease.* L. Packer and E. Cadenas, eds. M. Dekker, New York.

Hagen, T., Brown, L., and D. Jones. 1986. "Protection Against Paraquat-induced Injury by Exogenous Glutathione in Pulmonary Alveolar Type II Cells." *Biochemical Pharmacology.* 35:4537.

Jones, D., Hagen, T., Weber, R., et al. 1989. "Oral Administration of Glutathione Increases Plasma Glutathione Concentrations in Humans." *FASEB Journal.* 3:A1250.

Jones, D., Coates, R., Flagg, E., et al. 1992. "Glutathione in Foods Listed in the National Cancer Institute's Health Habits and History Food Frequency Questionnaire." *Nutriton and Cancer.* 17:57.

Kaplowitz, N. 1981. "The Importance and Regulation of Hepatic Glutathione." *Yale Journal of Biology and Medicine.* 54:497.

Lash, L., Hagen, T., and D. Jones. 1986. "Exogenous Glutathione Protects Intestinal Epithelial Cells from Oxidative Injury." *Porceedings of the National Academy of Sciences* (U.S.A.) 83:4641.

Mannervik, B., Carlberg, I., and K. Larson. 1989. "Glutathione: General Review of Mechanism of Action." In: *Glutathione. Chemical, Biochemical, and Medical Aspects.* Part A. Dolphin, Avramovic, and Poulson, eds., pp. 475–516, John Wiley and Sons, New York.

O'Neil, C., Halliwell, B., et al. 1994. "Aldehyde-Induced Protein Modification in Human Plasma: Protection by Glutathione and Dihydrolipoic Acid." *Journal of Laboratory and Clinical Medicine.* 124(3):359.

Suter, P., Domenighetti, G., et al. 1994. "N-Acetylcysteine Enhances Recovery From Acute Lung Injury in Man: a Randomized, Double-Blind, Placebo-Controlled Clinical Study." *Chest.* 105:190.

Alpha Lipoic Acid

Bashan, N., et al. 1993. "The Effect of Thioctic Acid on Glucose Transport." In: *The Role of Antioxidants in Diabetes.* F. Gries and K. Wessel, eds. pp. 221–229, PMI-Verlag-Gruppe.

Bast, A., and G. Haenen. 1988. "Interplay Between Lipoic Acid and Glutathione in the Protection against Microsomal Lipid Peroxidation." *Biochimica et Biophysica Acta.* 963:558.

Busse, E., Zimmer, G., et al. 1992. "Influence of Alpha Lipoic Acid on Intracellular Glutathione In Vitro and In Vivo." *Arzneimittelforschung.* 42:829.

Kagan, V., Shvedova, E., Serbinova, E., et al. 1992. "Dihydrolipoic Acid: A Universal Antioxidant Both in the Membrane and in the Aqueous Phase. Reduction of Peroxyl, Ascorbyl, and Chromanoxyl Radicals." *Biochemical Pharmacology.* 44(8):1637.

Packer, L., Witt, E., and H.J. Tritschler. 1995. "Alpha Lipic Acid as a Biological Antioxidant." *Free Radical Biology and Medicine.* 19(2):227.

Scholich, H., Murphy, M., and H. Sies. 1989. "Antioxidant Activity of Dihydrolipoate Against Microsomal Lipid Peroxidation, and its Dependance on Alpha Tocopherol." *Biochimica et Biophysica Acta.* 1001:256.

Suzuki, Y., et al. 1992. "Lipoate Prevents Glucose-Induced Protein Modifications." *Free Radical Research Communications.* 17:211.

Coenzyme Q10

Digiesi, V., Cantini, F., et al. 1994. "Coenzyme Q_{10} in Essential Hypertension." *Molecular Aspects of Medicine.* 15(suppl.):S257.

Folkers, K., Langsjoen, P., Nara, Y., Muratsu, K., Komorowski, J., Richardson, P. and Smith, T. 1988. "Biochemical Deficiencies of Coenzyme Q10 in HIV-Infection and Exploratory Treatment." *Biochemical and Biophysical Research Communications.* 153(2):888–896.

Folkers, K., Morita, M., and J. McRee. 1993. "The Activities of Coenzyme Q10 and Vitamin B6 for Immune Responses." *Biochemical and Biophysical Research Communications.* 193(1):88.

Folkers, K. 1993. "Heart failure is a Dominant Deficiency of Coenzyme Q10 and Challenges for Future Clinical Research on Coenzyme Q10." *Clinical Investigator.* 71:S51.

Greenberg, A., and W. Frishman. 1990. "Coenzyme Q10: A New Drug for Cardiovascular Disease." *Journal of Clinical Pharmacology.* 30:596.

Langsjoen, P., Willis, R., and K. Folkers. 1994. "Treatment of Essential Hypertension with Coenzyme Q_{10}." *Molecular Aspects of Medicine.* 15(suppl.):S265.

Lockwood, K., Moesgaard, S., et al. 1995. "Progress on Therapy of Breast Cancer with Vitamin Q_{10}, and the Regression of Metastases." *Biochemical and Biophysical Research Communications.* 212(1):172.

Tarui, S., Soga, F., et al. 1991. "Therapeutic Trials with Coenzyme Q10 for Mitochondrial Myopathies." In: *Mitochondrial Encephalomyopathies. Progress in Neuropathology.* DiMauro and Sato, eds. Vol 7. Raven Press, New York.

Thomas, S., Neuzil, J., and R. Stocker. 1996. "Co-Supplementation with Coenzyme Q_{10}, Prevents the Prooxidant Effect of Alpha Tocopherol and Increases the Resistance of LDL to Transition Metal-Dependent Oxidation Initiation." *Arteriosclerosis, Thrombosis and Vascular Biology.* 16:687.

Weber, C., Sejersgard, T., et al. 1994. "Antioxidant Effect of Dietary Coenzyme Q_{10} in Human Blood Plasma." *International Journal for Vitamin and Nutrition Research.* 64(4):311.

Pycnogenol

Gabor, D., et al. 1991. "Pycnogenol Inhibits Inflammation in a Dose-Dependant Manner." *Acta Physiologica Hungarica* (Budapest). 77:197.

Kuttan, R., Donnelly, P., et al. 1981. "Collagen Treated wtih Catechin Becomes Resistant to the Action of Mammalian Collagenase." *Experientia.* 37:221.

Masquelier, J. 1981. "Pycnogenols: Recent Advances in the Therapeutic Activity of Procyanidins." In: *Natural Products as Medicinal Agents.* J. Beal, E. Reinhard, eds. pp. 343–356, Hippokrates Verlag, Stuttgart.

Tixier, J., et al. 1984. "Evidence by In Vivo and In Vitro Studies That Binding of

Pycnogenols to Elastin Affects Its Rate of Degradation by Elastases." *Biochemical Pharmacology*. 33:3933.

Selenium

Anneren, G., Gebre-Medhin, M., and K. H. Gustavson. 1989. "Increased Plasma and Erythrocyte Glutathione Peroxidase Activity After Selenium Supplementation in Children with Down's Syndrome." *Acta Paediatrica Scandinavica*. 78:879–884.

Clark, L., Combs, G., et al. 1996. "Effects of Selenium Supplementation for Cancer Prevention in Patients with Carcinoma of the Skin." *Journal of the American Medical Association*. 276(24):1957.

Cowgill, U. M. 1983. "The Distribution of Selenium and Cancer Mortality in the Continental United States." *Biological Trace Element Research*. 5:345–361.

Delmas-Beauvieux, M.C., Peuchant, E., Couchouron, A., Constans, J., et al. 1996. "The Enzymatic Antioxidant System in Blood and Glutathione Status in Human Immunodeficiency Virus-Infected Patients: Effect of Supplementation with Selenium or Beta Carotene." *American Journal of Clinical Nutrition*. 64:101.

Diplock, A. 1993. "Indexes of Selenium Status in Human Populations." *American Journal of Clinical Nutrition*. 57:256S.

Horvath, P. M. and C. Ip. 1983. "Synergistic Effect of Vitamin E and Selenium in the Chemoprevention of Mammary Carcinogenesis in Rats." *Cancer Research*. 43:5335–5341.

Ip, C., and D. Lisk. 1995. "Efficacy of Cancer Prevention by High-Selenium Garlic is Primarily Dependant on the Action of Selenium." *Carcinogenesis*. 16(11):2649.

Lassen, K., Horder, M. 1994. "Selenium Status and the Effect of Organic and Inorganic Selenium Supplementation in a Group of Elderly People in Denmark." *Scandinavian Journal of Clinical and Laboratory Investigation*. 54(8):585.

Levander, O., and V. Morris. 1984. "Dietary Selenium Levels Needed to Maintain Balance in North American Adults Consuming Self-Selected Diets." *American Journal of Clinical Nutrition*. 39:809.

Luoma, P., Sotaniemi, E., et al., 1984. "Serum Selenium, Glutathione Peroxidase Activity and High Density Lipoprotein Cholesterol-effect of Selenium Supplementation." *Research Communications in Chemical Pathology and Pharmacology*. 46:469–472.

Salonen, J. T., Alfthan, G., Huttunen, J. K., and P. Puska. 1984. "Association Between Serum Selenium and the Risk of Cancer." *American Journal of Epidemiology*. 120:342–349.

Yang, G., Xia, Y. 1995. "Studies on Human Dietary Requirements and Safe Range of Dietary Intakes of Selenium in China, and Their Application in the Prevention of Related Endemic Disease." *Biomedical and Environmental Sciences*. 8(3):187.

Folate

Boushey, C., et al. 1995. "A Quantitative Assessment of Plasma Homocysteine as a Risk Factor for Vascular Disease." *Journal of the American Medical Association*. 274:1049.

Glynn, S., and D. Albanes. 1994. "Folate and Cancer. A Review of the Literature." *Nutrition and Cancer*. 22:101.

Jaques, P., Bostom, A., et al. 1996. "Relation Between Folate Status, a Common Mutation in Methylenetetrahydrofolate Reductase, and Plasma Homocysteine Concentrations." *Circulation*. 93(1):7.

Kirke, P., Daly, L., and J. Elwood. 1992. "A Randomized Trial of Low-Dose Folic Acid to Prevent Neural Tube Defects: the Irish Vitamin Study Group." *Archives of Disease in Childhood*. 67:1442.

Mason, J., and T. Levesque. 1996. "Folate: Effects on Carcinogenesis and the Potential for Cancer Chemoprevention." *Oncology.* 10(11):1727.
Riggs, K., Spiro, A., et al. 1996. "Relations of Vitamin B-12, Vitamin B-6, Folate, and Homocysteine to Cognitive Performance in the Normative Aging Study." *American Journal of Clinical Nutrition.* 63:306.

Zinc
Bogden, J., Oleske, J., et al. 1987. "Zinc and Immunocompetence in the Elderly: Baseline Data on Zinc Nutriture and Immunity in Unsupplemented Subjects." *American Journal of Clinical Nutrition.* 46:101.
Gladstone, J., and R. Recco. 1976. "Host Factors and Infectious Diseases in the Elderly." *Medical Clinics of North America.* 60:1225.
Hadden, J. 1995. "The Treatment of Zinc Deficiency Is an Immunotherapy." *International Journal of Immunopharmacology.* 17(9):697.
Lee, D., Ananda, S., et al. 1993. "Homeostasis of Zinc in Marginal Human Zinc Deficiency: Role of Absorption and Endogenous Excretion of Zinc." *Journal of Laboratory and Clinical Medicine.* 122:549.
Mossad, S., Macknin, M., et al. 1996. "Zinc Gluconate Lozenges for Treating the Common Cold." *Annals of Internal Medicine.* 125(2):81.
Prasad, A. 1996. "Zinc Deficiency in Women, Infants, and Children." *Journal of the American College of Nutrition.* 15(2):113.
Walsh, C., Sandstead, H., et al. 1994. "Zinc: Health Effects and Research Priorities for the 1990s." *Environmental Health Perspectives.* 102:5.

Phosphatidylcholine
Buzzelli, G., et al. 1993. "A Pilot Study on the Liver Protective Effect of Silybin-Phosphatidylcholine Complex (IdB 1016) in Chronic, Active Hepatitis." *International Journal of Clinical Pharmacology, Therapy, and Toxicology* (München). 31(9):456.
Hantak, I., et al. 1990. "Essential Phospholipids in the Treatment of Chronic Infection with the Hepatitis-B Virus." *Vnitrni Lekarstvi (Internal Medicine).* 36:1164. (Translated from the Slovak.)
Jenkins, P., et al. 1982. "Use of Polyunsaturated Phosphatidylcholine in HBsAg Negative Chronic Active Hepatitis: Results of Prospective Double-Blind Controlled Trial." *Liver.* 2:77.
Kalab, M., and J. Cervinka. 1983. "Essential Phospholipids in the Treatment of Cirrhosis of the Liver." *Cas Lek ces (Czech Journal of Medicine).* 122:266. (In Slovak, with English summary.)
Kneuchel, F. 1979. "Double-Blind Study in Patients with Alcohol-Toxic Fatty Liver." *Medizinische Welt.* 30(11):411.
Lieber, C., et al. 1994. "Phosphatidylcholine Protects against Fibrosis and Cirrhosis in the Baboon." *Gastroenterology.* 106:152.
Schuller Perez, A., and San Martin, F. 1985. "Controlled Study Using Multiply-Unsaturated Phosphatidylcholine in Comparison with Placebo in the Case of Alcoholic Liver Steatosis." *Medizinische Welt.* 72(36):517.

Omega-3 Fatty Acids
Chen, C., Wong, J., Lee, N., Chan-Ho, M., Lau, J. T., and M. Fung. 1993. "The Shatin Community Mental Health Survey in Hong Kong II. Major Findings." *Archives of General Psychiatry.* 50:125–133.
Daviglus, M, Stamler, J., et al. 1997. "Fish Consumption and the Thirty-Year Risk of Fatal Myocardial Infarction." *New England Journal of Medicine.* 336:1046.

Dyerberg, J., et al. 1978. "Eicosapentaenoic Acid and Prevention of Thrombosis and Atherosclerosis." *Lancet.* 2:117.

Hibbeln, J. R. and N. Salem. 1995. "Dietary Polyunsaturated Fatty Acids and Depression: When Cholesterol Does Not Satisfy." *American Journal of Clinical Nutrition.* 62:1–9.

Kremer, J. 1991. "Clinical Studies of Omega-3 Fatty Acid Supplementation in Patients with Rheumatoid Arthritis." *Rheumatic Diseases Clinics of North America.* 17:391.

Nair, S.S.D., Leitch, J., et al. 1997. "Prevention of Cardiac Arrhythmia by Dietary (n-3) Polyunsaturated Fatty Acids and Their Mechanism of Action." *Journal of Nutrition.* 127:383.

Pauletto, P., Puato, M., et al. 1996. "Blood Pressure and Atherogenic Lipoprotein Profiles of Fish-Diet and Vegetarian Villagers in Tanzania: The Lugalawa Study." *Lancet.* 348:784.

Rose, D., Connolly, J., and X. Liu. 1994. "Diet and Breast Cancer." *American Institute for Cancer Research.* pp. 83–91, Plenum Press, New York.

Welsch, C., 1992. "Relationship Between Dietary Fat and Experimental Mammary Tumorigenesis: A Review and Critique." *Cancer Research.* 52:2040S.

Aspirin

Antiplatelet Trialist's Collaboration. 1994. "Collaborative Overview of Randomized Trials of Antiplatelet Therapy. I. Prevention of Death, Myocardial Infarction, and Stroke by Prolonged Antiplatelet Therapy in Various Categories of Patients." *British Medical Journal.* 308:81.

Breitner, J., Gau, B., et al. 1994. "Inverse Association of Antiinflammatory Treatments and Alzheimer's Disease." *Neurology.* 44:227.

Heath, C., Thun, M., et al. 1994. "Nonsteroidal Antiinflammatory Drugs and Human Cancer." *Cancer.* 74:2885.

Hennekens, C. 1997. "Update on Aspirin in the Primary and Secondary Prevention of Cardiovascular Disease." *Hospital Medicine.* January.

McGeer, P., et al. 1996. "Arthritis and Antiinflammatory Agents as Possible Protective Factors for Alzheimer's Disease." *Neurology.* 47:425.

Rogers, J., Kirby, L., et al. 1993. "Clinical Trial of Indomethacin in Alzheimer's Disease." *Neurology.* 43:1609.

Schatzkin, A., and G. Kelloff. 1995. "Chemo- and Dietary Prevention of Colorectal Cancer." *European Journal of Cancer.* 31A(no.7/8):1198.

Steering Committee of the Physician's Health Study Research Group. 1989. "Final Report on the Aspirin Component of the Ongoing Physicians Health Study." *New England Journal of Medicine.* 321:129.

Stewart, W., et al. 1997. "Risk of Alzheimer's Disease and Duration of NSAID Use." *Neurology* 48:262.

Chapter Ten: Muscle and Energy Tools I: Hormones

DHEA

Araneo, B., Dowell, T., et al. 1995. "DHEAS as an Effective Vaccine Adjuvant in Elderly Humans." Proof of Principles. *Annals of the New York Academy of Sciences.* Vol. 774. pp. 232–248.

Barrett-Connor, E., Khaw, K.T., and S.C. Yen. 1986. "A Prospective Study of Dehydroepiandrosterone Sulfate, Mortality, and Cardiovascular Disease." *New England Journal of Medicine.* 315:1519.

Belanger, A., Candas, B., et al. 1994. "Changes in Serum Concentrations of Conjugated and Unconjugated Steroids in 40- to 80-Year-Old Men." *Journal of Clinical Endocrinology and Metabolism.* 79(4):1086.

Bergeron R, de Montigny, C., and G. Debonnel. 1996. "Potentiation of Neuronal NMDA Response Induced by Dehydroepiandrosterone and Its Suppression by Progesterone: Effects Mediated Via Sigma Receptors." *Journal of Neuroscience.* 16(3):1193.

Bologa, L., Sharma, J., and E. Roberts. 1987. "Dehydroepiandrosterone and Its Sulfated Derivative Reduce Neuronal Death and Enhance Astrocyte Differentiation in Brain Cell Cultures." *Journal of Neuroscience Research.* 17:225.

Bonnet, K. 1990. "Cognitive Effects of DHEA Replacement Therapy." In: *The Biological Role of DHEA.* M. Kalami and W. Regelson, eds. pp. 65–79, Walter de Gruyter, New York.

Casson, P., Straughn, A., et al. 1996. "Delivery of Dehydroepiandrosterone to Premenopausal Women: Effects of Micronization and Nonoral Administration." *American Journal of Obstetrics and Gynecology.* 174:649.

Diamond, P., Cusan, L., et al. 1996. "Metabolic Effects of 12-Month Percutaneous Dehydroepiandrosterone Replacement Therapy in Post-Menopausal Women." *Journal of Endocrinology.* 150:S43.

Flood, J., and E. Roberts. 1988. "Dehydroepiandrosterone Sulfate Improves Memory in Aging Mice." *Brain Research.* 448:178.

Freiss, E., Trachsel, L., et al. 1995. "DHEA Administration Increases Rapid Eye Movement Sleep and EEG Power in the Sigma Frequency." *American Journal of Physiology.* 268:E107.

Jacobson, M., et al. 1991. "Decreased Serum Dehydroepiandrosterone is Associated with an Increased Progression of Human Immunodeficiency Virus Infection in Men with CD4 Cell Counts of 200–499." *Journal of Infectious Diseases.* 164:864.

Khorram, O., Vu, L., and S.S.C. Yen. 1997. "Activation of Immune Function by Dehydroepiandrosterone (DHEA) in Age-Advanced Men." *Journal of Gerontology.* 52A(1):M1–M7.

Lane, M., Ingram, D., et al. 1997. "Dehydroepiandrosterone Sulfate: A Biomarker of Primate Aging Slowed by Caloric Restriction." *Journal of Clinical Endocrinology and Metabolism.* 82(7):2093.

Loria, R., et al. 1996. "Regulation of the Immune Response by Dehydroepiandrosterone and Its Metabolites." *Journal of Endocrinology.* 150:S209.

Mitchell, L., Sprecher, D., et al. 1993. "Evidence for an Association Between Dehydroepiandrosterone Sulfate and Non-Fatal, Premature Myocardial Infarction in Males." *Circulation.* 89:89.

Morales, A., Nolan, J., et al. 1994. "Effects of Replacement Dose of Dehydroepiandrosterone in Men and Women of Advancing Age." *Journal of Clinical Endocrinology and Metabolism.* 78(6):1360.

Nestler, J. Clore, J., et al. 1987. The Effects of Hyperinsulinemia on Serum Testosterone, Progesterone, Dehydroepiandrosterone Sulfate, and Cortisol Levels in Normal Women and in Women with Hyperandrogenism, Insulin Resistance, and Acanthosis Nigricans. *Journal of Clinical Endocrinology and Metabolism.* 64:180.

Thomas, G., et al. 1994. "Serum Dehydroepiandrosterone Sulfate Levels as an Individual marker." *Journal of Clinical Endocrinology and Metabolism.* 79(5):1273.

Van Vollenhoven, R., Engleman, E., and J. McGuire. 1994. "An Open Study of Dehydroepiandrosterone in Systemic Lupus Erythematous." *Arthritis and Rheumatism.* 37(9):1305.

Watson, R., et al. 1996. "Dehydroepiandrosterone and the Diseases of Aging." *Drugs and Aging.* 9(4):274.

Wolkowitz, O., Reus, V., et al. 1997. "Dehydroepiandrosterone (DHEA) Treatment of Depression." *Biological Psychiatry.* 41:311.

Yen, S.S.C., Morales, A., and O. Khorram. 1995. "Replacement of DHEA in Aging Men and Women. Potential Remedial Effects." *Annals of the New York Academy of Sciences.* Vol. 774. pp. 128–142.

Growth Hormone

Auernhammer C., et al. 1995. "Effects of Growth Hormone and Insulin-Like Growth Factor I on the Immune System." *European Journal of Endocrinology.* 133:635.

Chapman, I., Bach, M., et al. 1996. "Stimulation of the Growth Hormone (GH)-Insulin-Like Growth Factor I Axis by Daily Oral Administration of a GH Secretogogue (MK-677) in Healthy Elderly Subjects." *Journal of Clinical Endocrinology and Metabolism.* 81(12):4249.

Gelato, M. 1996. "Aging and Immune Function: A Possible Role for Growth Hormone." *Hormone Research.* 45:46.

Johannsson, G., Marin, P., et al. 1997. "Growth Hormone Treatment of Abdominally Obese Men Reduces Abdominal Fat Mass, Improves Glucose and Lipoprotein Metabolism, and Reduces Diastolic Blood Pressure." *Journal of Clinical Endocrinology and Metabolism.* 82(3):727.

Johnston, D., and B. Bengtsson. 1993. "Workshop Report: The Effects of Growth Hormone and Growth Hormone-Deficiency on Lipids and the Cardiovascular System." *Acta Endocrinologica.* 128(suppl.2):69.

Kelijman, M. 1991. "Age-Related Alterations of the GH/Insulin-Like Growth Factor 1 Axis." *Journal of the American Geriatric Society.* 39:295.

Khorram, O., Laughlin, G., and S.S.C. Yen. 1997. "Endocrine and Metabolic Effects of Long-Term Administration of [Nle27] Growth Hormone-Releasing Hormone-(1–29)-NH2 in Age-Advanced Men and Women." *Journal of Clinical Endocrinology and Metabolism.* 82(5):1472.

Rudman, D. 1985. "Growth Hormone, Body Composition, and Aging." *Journal of the American Geriatric Society.* 33:800.

Rudman, D., Feller, A.G. et al. 1990. "Effects of Human GH in Men Over 60 Years Old." *New England Journal of Medicine.* 323:1.

Melatonin

Cohen, M., Josimovich, J., and A. Brezinski. 1995. *Melatonin: From Contraception to Breast Cancer Prevention.* Sheba Press (Maryland).

Honma, K. et al. 1992. "Effects of Vitamin B12 on Plasma Melatonin Rhythm in Humans: Increased Light Sensitivity Phase Advances the Circadian Clock." *Experientia.* 48:716.

Iguchi, H., Kato, K., and H. Ibayashi. 1982. "Age-Dependant Reduction in Serum Melatonin Concentrations in Healthy Human Subjects." *Journal of Clinical Endocrinology and Metabolism.* 55:27.

Lewy, A., Wehr, T., and F. Goodwin. 1980. "Light Suppresses Melatonin Secretion in Humans." *Science.* Volume 210.

Maestroni, G., et al. 1988. "Pineal Melatonin, Its Fundamental Immunoregulatory Role in Aging and Cancer." *Annals of the New York Academy of Sciences.* 521:140.

McIntyre, I., Norman, T., and G. Burrows. 1990. "Melatonin Supersensitivity to Dim Light in Seasonal Affective Disorder." *Lancet.* 335:488.

Muller-Weiland, D., Behnke, D., and W. Krone. 1994. "Melatonin Inhibits LDL-Receptor Activity and Cholesterol Synthesis in Freshly Isolated Human Mononuclear Leukocytes." *Biochemical Biophysical Research Communications.* 203(1):416.

Neri, B., et al. 1995. "Effects of Melatonin Administration on Cytokine Production in Patients with Advanced Solid Tumors." *Oncology Reports.* 2:45.

Poeggeler, B., Reiter, R., et al. 1993. "Melatonin, Hydroxyl Radical-Mediated Oxida-tive Damage, and Aging: A Hypothesis." *Journal of Pineal Research*. 14:151.

Rao, M., et al. 1990. "The Influence of Phototherapy on Serotonin and Melatonin in Non-Seasonal Depression." *Pharmacopsychiatry*. 23:155.

Reiter, R.J., et al. 1994. "The Role of Melatonin in the Pathophysiology of Oxygen Radical Damage." In: *Advances in Pineal Research*. Vol. 8. M. Moller and P. Pevet, eds. John Libby and Co., London.

Reiter, R.J., Pablos, M.I., Agapito, T., and J. Guerrero. 1996. "Melatonin in the Context of the Free Radical Theory of Aging." In: *Pharmacological Interven-tion in Aging and Age-Associated Disorders*. K. Kitani, A. Aoba, and S. Goto, eds. *Annals of the New York Academy of Sciences*. Vol 786 pp. 362–378.

Tan, D.X., Poeggeler, B., and R. Reiter. 1993. "The Pineal Hormone Melatonin Inhibits DNA-Adduct Formation Induced by the Chemical Carcinogen Safrole In Vivo." *Cancer Letters*. 70:65–71.

Vijayalaxmi, B., Reiter, R., et al. 1995. "Melatonin Protects Human Blood Lympho-cytes from Radiation-Induced Chromosome Damage." *Mutation Research*. 346(1):23.

Wright, K., et al. 1995. "Effects of Caffeine, Bright Light, and Their Combination on Night-Time Melatonin and Temperature During Two Nights of Sleep Depri-vation." *Sleep Research*. 24:458.

Chapter Eleven: Muscle and Energy Tools II: Physical Exercise

American College of Sports Medicine. 1990. "The Recommended Quantity and Quality of Exercise for Developing and Maintaining Cardiorespiratory and Mus-cular Fitness in Healthy Adults." *Medicine and Science in Sports and Exer-cise*. 22(2):265.

Benjamin, H., et al. 1988. "Effect of Voluntary Exercise on Mamary Tumor Develop-ment." *FASEB Journal*. 2:A1191 (abstr.).

Boutcher, S., and D. Landers. 1988. "The Effects of Vigorous Exercise on Anxiety, Heart Rate, and Alpha Activity of Runners and Non-Runners." *Psychophysiol-ogy*. 23:696.

Crist, D., et al. 1989. "Physical Exercise Increases Natural Cellular-Mediated Tumor Cytotoxicity in Elderly Women." *Gerontology*. 35:66.

Despres, J., Tremblay, A., et al. 1988. "Physical Training and Changes in Regional Adipose Tissue Distribution." *Acta Medica Scandinavica*. 723:205 (suppl.).

Dishman, R. 1992. "Psychological Effects of Exercise for Disease Resistance and Health Promotion." In: *Exercise and Disease*. R. Watson and M. Eisinger, eds. CRC Press, Boca Raton, Florida.

Fiatarone, M., Morley, J., et al. 1989. "The Effect of Exercise on Natural Killer Cell Activity in Young and Old Subjects." *Journal of Gerontology*. 44:M37.

Frederiksson, M., Bengtsson, N., et al. 1989. "Colon Cancer, Physical Activity, and Occupational Exposures." *Cancer*. 63:1838.

Frisch, R., Wyshak, G., et al. 1985. "Lower Prevalence of Breast Cancer and Cancers of the Reproductive System among Former College Atheltes, Compared to Non-Athletes." *British Journal of Cancer*. 52:885.

Frisch, R., Wyshak, G., et al. 1989. "Lower Prevalence of Non-Reproductive System Cancers among Female Former College Athletes." *Medicine and Science in Sports and Exercise*. 21:250.

Goran, M., and E. Poehlman. 1992. "The Role of Physical Activity in the Develop-ment of Childhood Obesity." In: *Exercise and Disease*. R. Watson and M. Eisinger, eds. CRC Press, Boca Raton, Florida.

Hagberg, J. 1990. "Exercise, Fitness, and Hypertension." In: *Exercise, Fitness, and Health*. Bouchard, Shepard, et al., eds. Human Kinetics Publishers, Champaign, Illinois.

Haskell, W. 1985. "The Influence of Exercise Training on Plasma Lipids and Lipoproteins in Health and Disease." *Acta Medica Scandinavica*. 711:25.

Hill, R., et al. 1993. "The Impact of Long-term Exercise Training on Psychological Function in Older Adults." *Journal of Gerontology*. 48:P12.

Hyatt, R., et al. 1990. "Association of Muscle Strength with Functional Status of Elderly People." *Age Ageing*. 19:330.

King, A., et al. 1997. "Moderate Intensity Exercise and Self-Rated Quality of Sleep in Older Adults." *Journal of the American Medical Association*. 277(1):32.

Keast, D., et al. 1988. "Exercise and the Immune Response." *Sports Medicine*. 5:248.

Kushi, L., et al. 1997. "Physical Activity and Mortality in Post-Menopausal Women." *Journal of the American Medical Association*. 277(16):1287.

Leon, A., Connett, J., et al. 1987. "Leisure Time Physical Activity Levels and Risk of Coronary Heart Disease and Death: the Multiple Risk Factor Intervention Trial." *Journal of the American Medical Association*. 258:2388.

Martinsen, E. 1987. "The Role of Aerobic Exercise in the Treatment of Depression." *Stress Medicine*. 3:93.

Masuhara, M., et al. 1987. "Influence of Exercise on Leukocyte Count and Size." *Journal of Sports Medicine*. 27:285.

Mazzeo, R., and I. Nasrullah. 1992. "Exercise and Age-Related Decline in Immune Function." In: *Exercise and Disease*. R. Watson and M. Eisinger, eds. CRC Press, Boca Raton, Florida.

McCartney, N., et al. 1996. "A Longitudinal Trial of Weight Training in the Elderly: Continued Improvements in Year II." *Journal of Gerontology*. 51A(6):B425.

Miller, J., et al. 1994. "Strength Training Increases Insulin Sensitivity in Healthy 50- to 65-Year-Old Men." *Journal of Applied Physiology*. 77:1122.

Moore, K. 1997. Results of Exercise/Depression Study Presented at April 1997 Meeting of Society of Behavioral Medicine.

Moran, M., et al. 1988. "Sleep Disorders in the Elderly." *American Journal of Psychiatry*. 145:1369.

Moran, M., and N. Azrin. 1988. "Behavioral and Cognitive Treatments of Geriatric Insomnia." *Journal of Consulting and Clinical Psychology*. 56:748.

Neeper, S., Gomez-Pinilla, F., et al. 1995. "Exercise and Brain Neurotrophins." *Nature*. 373:109.

Nehlsen-Cannarella, S., et al. 1990. "The Effects of Moderate Exercise Training on Immune Response." *Medicine and Science in Sports and Exercise*. 23:64.

Nicklas, B., Ryan, A., et al. 1995. "Testosterone, Growth Hormone, and IGF Responses to Acute and Chronic Resistive Exercise in Men aged 55 to 70 years." *International Journal of Sports Medicine*. 16:445.

Packer, L. 1986. "Oxygen Radicals and Antioxidants in Endurance Exercise." In: *Biochemical Aspects of Physical Exercise*. Benzi, Packer, Siliprandi, eds. pp. 73–92. Elsevier Publishers, Amsterdam.

Petruzzello, S., Landers, D., et al. 1991. "Meta Analysis on the Anxiety-Reducing Effects of Acute and Chronic Exercise." *Sports Medicine*. 11:143.

Rogers, R., Meyers, J., et al. 1990. "After Reaching Retirement Age, Physical Activity Sustains Cerebral Perfusion and Cognition." *Journal of the American Geriatric Society*. 38:123.

Ryan, A., et al. 1996. "Resistive Training Increases Insulin Action in Postmenopausal Women." *Journal of Gerontology*. 51A(5):M199.

Starr, J., et al. 1993. "Blood Pressure and Cognitive Function in Healthy Old People." *Journal of the American Geriatric Society*. 41:753.

Sumida, S., et al. 1989. "Exercise-Induced Lipid Peroxidation and Leakage Enzymes

Before and After Vitamin E Supplementation." *International Journal of Biochemistry.* 21:835.

Thune, I., Brenn, T., et al. 1997. "Physical Activity and the Risk of Breast Cancer." *New England Journal of Medicine.* 336(18):1269.

Tinetti, M., et al. 1988. "Risk Factors or Falls among Elderly Persons Living in the Community." *New England Journal of Medicine.* 319:1701.

Tipton, C. 1991. "Exercise, Training, and Hypertension: an Update." *Exercise and Sports Sciences Review.* 19:447.

Tonind, L., Helzer, J., et al. 1984. "Lifetime Prevalence of Specific Psychiatric Disorders in Three Sites." *Archives of General Psychiatry.* 41:949.

Tonino, R. 1989. "Effect of Physical Training on the Insulin Resistance of Aging." *American Journal of Physiology.* 256:E352.

Vranic, M., and D. Wasserman. 1990. "Exercise, Fitness, and Diabetes." In: *Exercise, Fitness, and Health; A Consensus of Current Knowledge.* Bouchard, Shephard, et al., eds. Human Kinetics Publishers, Champaign, Illinois.

Whittemore, A., Wu-Williams, A., et al. 1990. "Diet, Physical Activity, and Colorectal Cancer among Chinese in North America and China." *Journal of the National Cancer Institute.* 82:915.

Chapter Twelve: Muscle and Energy Tools III: Diet

Beard, J. 1993. "Are We at Risk for Heart Disease because of Normal Iron Status?" *Nutrition Reviews.* 51(4):112.

Bjorntorp, P., et al. 1988. "Health Implications of Regional Obesity." *Acta Medica Scandinavica.* 723:1 (suppl.).

Bostom, A.G., Cupples, L.A., Jenner, J.L., et al. 1996. "Elevated Plasma Lipoprotein(a) and Coronary Heart Disease in Men Aged 55 years and Younger." *Journal of the American Medical Association.* 276(7):544.

Byers, T. 1993. "Dietary Trends in the United States." *Cancer.* 72:1015.

Carroll, K., and E. Kurowska. 1995. "Soy Consumption and Cholesterol Reduction: A Review of Animal and Human Studies." *Journal of Nutrition.* 125:594S.

Chung, M., et al. 1992. "Protection of DNA Damage by Dietary Restriction." *Journal of Free Radicals in Biology and Medicine.* 12:523.

Colditz, G. 1992. "Economic Costs of Obesity." *American Journal of Clinical Nutrition.* 55:503S.

Ely, D. 1997. "Overview of Dietary Sodium Effects on and Interactions with Cardiovascular and Neuroendocrine Functions." *American Journal of Clinical Nutrition.* 65(suppl.):594S.

Fernandes, G., Friend, P., Yunis, E.J., and R.A. Good. 1978. "Influence of Dietary Restriction on Immunological Function and Renal Disease in (NZBXNZW)F_1 Mice." *Proceedings of the National Academy of Sciences* (U.S.A.). 75:1500–1504.

Gotto, A. 1997. "Cholesterol Management in Theory and Practice." *Circulation.* 96(12):4424.

Jeppesen, J. Schaaf, P., et al. 1997. "Effects of Low-Fat, High-Carbohydrate Diets on Risk Factors for Ischemic Heart Disease in Postmenopausal Women." *American Journal of Clinical Nutrition.* 65:1027.

Kannel, W.B. 1995. "Range of Serum Cholesterol Values in the Population Developing Coronary Artery Disease." *American Journal of Cardiology.* 76:69C.

Keichl, S., et al. 1997. "Body Iron Stores and the Risk of Atherosclerosis." *Circulation.* 96:3300.

Kucamarksi, R., Flegal, K., et al. 1994. "Increasing Prevalence of Overweight among U.S. Adults." *Journal of the American Medical Association.* 272:205.

Maher, V., Brown, G., et al. 1995. "Effects of Lowering LDL Cholesterol on the Cardiovascular Risk of Apolipoprotein A." *Journal of the American Medical Association.* 274:1771.

Manson, J., and G. Faich. 1996. "Pharmacotherapy for Obesity: Do the Benefits Outweigh the Risk?" *New England Journal of Medicine.* 335(9):659.

Masaro, E., and S. Austad. 1996. "The Evolution of the Antiaging Action of Dietary Restriction: A Hypothesis." *Journal of Gerontology.* 51A(6):B387.

Mensink, R., Zock, P., et al. 1992. "Effect of Dietary Cis and Trans Fatty Acids on Serum Lipoprotein A Levels in Humans." *Journal of Lipid Research.* 33:1493.

Meyers, D., et al. 1997. "Possible Association of a Reduction in Cardiovascular Events with Blood Donation." *Heart.* 78(2):188–193.

Pitsikas, N., Garofalo, P., Manfridi, A., Zanotti, A., and S. Algeri. 1991. "Effect of Life-Long Hypocaloric Diet on Discrete Memory of the Senescent Rat." *Aging.* 3:147–152.

Potter, S.M. 1995. "Overview of Proposed Mechanisms for Hypocholesterolemic Effect of Soy." *Journal of Nutrition.* 125:606S.

Salmeron, J., Manson, J., et al. 1997. "Dietary Fiber, Glycemic Load, and Risk of Non-Insulin Dependent Diabetes Mellitus in Women." *Journal of the American Medical Association.* 277(6):472.

Salonen, J., Nyyssonen, K., et al. 1992. "High Stored Iron Levels Are Associated with Excess Risk of Myocardial Infarction in Eastern Finnish Men." *Circulation.* 86(3):803.

Sohol, R., and R. Weindruch. 1996. "Oxidative Stress, Caloric Restriction, and Aging." *Science.* 273:59.

Stevens, R., Jones, D., et al. 1988. "Body Iron Stores and the Risk of Cancer." *New England Journal of Medicine.* 319(16):1047.

Takata, H., Ishi, T., et al. 1987. "Influence of Major Histocompatibility Complex Region Genes on Human Longevity among Okinawan Japanese Centenarians and Nonagenarians." *Lancet.* 2:824.

Tobian, L. 1997. "Dietary Sodium Chloride and Potassium Have Effects on the Pathophysiology of Hypertension in Humans and Animals." *American Journal of Clinical Nutrition.* 65(suppl.):606S.

Walford, R., et al. 1992. "The Calorically Restricted Lowfat Nutrient Dense Diet in Biosphere II Significantly Lowers Blood Glucose, Total Leukocyte Count, Cholesterol, and Blood Pressure in Humans." *Proceedings of the National Academy of Sciences* (U.S.A.). 89(23):11533.

Warshafsky, S., et al. 1993. "Effect of Garlic on Total Serum Cholesterol: a Meta-Analysis." *Annals of Internal Medicine.* 119:599.

Weindruch, R., Albanes, D., and D. Kritchevsky. 1991. "The Role of Calories and Caloric Restriction in Carcinogenesis." *Hematology/Oncology Clinics of North America.* 5(1):79–89.

Weindruch, R., and R.L. Walford. 1988. *The Retardation of Aging and Disease by Dietary Restriction.* Charles C. Thomas Publishers, Springfield, Illinois.

Yu, B.P., Laganiere, S., and J.W. Kim. 1989. "Influence of Life-Prolonging Food Restriction on Membrane Lipid Peroxidation and Antioxidant States." In: *Oxygen Radicals in Biology and Medicine.* Simic, Taylor, Ward, and von Sonntag, eds. pp. 1067–1073, Plenum Press, New York.

Chapter Thirteen: Young and Sexy Tools I: Hormones

Estrogen

Andrews, W. 1995. "The Transitional Years and Beyond." *Obstetrics and Gynecology*. 85:1.

Bancroft, J., and E. Cawood. 1997. "Androgens and the Menopause: a Study of 40–60-Year-Old Women." *Clinical Endocrinology*. 45:577.

Cavley, J., Cummings, S., et al. 1990. "Prevalence and Determinants of Estrogen Replacement Therapy in Elderly Women." *American Journal of Obstetrics and Gynecology*. 163:1438.

Colditz, G.A., Egan, K.M., and M.J. Stampfer. 1993. "Hormone Replacement Therapy and Risk of Breast Cancer: Results from Epidemiological Studies." *American Journal of Obstetrics and Gynecology*. 168:1473.

Colditz, G.A., Hankinson, S.E., Hunter, D.J., et al. 1995. "The Use of Estrogens and Progestins and the Risk of Breast Cancer in Post-Menopausal Women." *New England Journal of Medicine*. 332:1589.

Dunn, L., et al. 1997. "Does Estrogen Prevent Skin Aging?" *Archives of Dermatology*. 133:339.

Ewertz, M. 1988. "Influence of Non-Contraceptive Exogenous and Endogenous Sex Hormones on Breast Cancer Risk in Denmark." *International Journal of Cancer*. 42:832.

Grodstein, F., Stampfer, M.J., et al. 1997. "Post-Menopausal Hormone Therapy and Mortality." *New England Journal of Medicine*. 336(25):1769.

Hammond, C., 1996. "Menopause and Hormone Replacement Therapy: An Overview." *Obstetrics and Gynecology*. 87:2S.

Tranquilli, A., Mazzani, L., et al. 1995. "Transdermal Estradiol and Medroxyprogesterone Acetate in Hormone-Replacement Therapy Are Both Antioxidants." *Gynecological Endocrinology*. 9:137.

Wild, R. 1996. "Estrogen: Effects on the Cardiovascular Tree." *Obstetrics and Gynecology*. 87(2):27S.

The Writing Group for the PEPI Trial. 1996. "Effects of Hormone Replacement Therapy on Endometrial Histology in Post-Menopausal Women." *Journal of the American Medical Association*. 275(5):370.

Testosterone

Bardin, C., et al. 1991. Special article. "Androgens: Risks and Benefits." *Journal of Clinical Endocrinology and Metabolism*. 73(1):4.

Bhasin, S., Storer, T., et al. 1996. "The Effects of Supraphysiologic Doses of Testosterone on Muscle Size and Strength in Normal Men." *New England Journal of Medicine*. 335(1):1.

Carini, C., Zini, D., et al. 1990. "Effects of Androgen Treatment in Impotent Men with Normal and Low Levels of Free Testosterone." *Archives of Sexual Behavior*. 19:223.

Gray, A., Feldman, H., et al. 1991. "Age, Disease, and Changing Sex Hormone levels in Middle-Aged Men: Results of the Massachusetts Male-Aging Study." *Journal of Clinical Endocrinology and Metabolism*. 73:1016.

Grinspoon, S., Corcoran, C., et al. 1996. "Loss of Lean Body and Muscle Mass Correlates with Androgen Levels in Hypogonadal Men with Acquired Immunodeficiency Syndrome and Wasting." *Journal of Clinical Endocrinology and Metabolism*. 81(11):4051.

Janowsky, J., Oviatt, S., and E. Orwoll. 1994. "Testosterone Influences Spatial Cognition in Older Men." *Behavioral Neuroscience*. 108(2):325.

Kaiser, F., Viosca, S., et al. 1988. "Impotence and Aging: Clinical and Hormonal Factors." *Journal of the American Geriatric Society.* 36:511.

Kerr, J., Allore, R., et al. 1995. "Distribution and Hormonal Regulation of Androgen Receptor (AR) and AR Messenger RNA in the Rat Hippocampus." *Endocrinology.* 136:3213.

Kley, H., Solbach, H., et al. 1979. "Testosterone Decrease and Estrogen Increase in Male Patients with Obesity." *Acta Endocrinologica.* 91:553.

Morley, J., Perry, H., et al. 1993. "Effects of Testosterone Replacement in Old Hypogonadal Males. A Preliminary Study." *Journal of the American Geriatric Society.* 41:149.

Morley, J. (S. Boschert). 1994. "Testosterone Loss May Affect Memory in Elderly Men." *Internal Medicine News and Cardiology News.* Issue of September 1. Page 8.

O'Carroll, R., and J. Bancroft. 1984. "Testosterone Therapy for Low Sexual Interest and Erectile Dysfunction in Men. A Controlled Study." *British Journal of Psychiatry.* 145:146.

Phillips, G., Pinkernell, B., and T.Y. Yjing. 1993. "The Association of Hypotestoeronemia with Coronary Artery Disease in Men." *Arteriosclerosis and Thrombosis.* 14:701.

Rubin, R., Poland, R., and I. Lesser. 1989. "Neuroendocrine Aspects of Primary Endogenous Depression. VIII. Pituitary Gonadal Axis Activity in Male Patients and Matched Control Subjects." *Psychoneuroendocrinology.* 14:217.

Tenover, J., Matsumoto, A., et al. 1987. "The Effects of Aging in Normal Men on Bioavailable Testosterone and Luteinizing Hormone Secretion: Response to Clomiphene Citrate. *Journal of Clinical Endocrinology and Metabolism.* 65:1118.

Tenover, J. 1992. "Effects of Testosterone Supplementation in the Aging Male." *Journal of Clinical Endocrinology and Metabolism.* 75(4):1092.

Vermeulen, A. 1991. "The Aging Male." *Journal of Clinical Endocrinology and Metabolism.* 73:221.

Yesavage, J., Davidson, J., et al. 1985. "Plasma Testosterone Levels, Depression, Sexuality and Age." *Biological Psychiatry.* 20:199.

Chapter Fifteen: Looking Good Tools I: Skin *Don'ts*

Mackie, B., et al. 1987. "Melanoma and Dietary Lipids." *Nutrition and Cancer.* 9:219.

Miyachi, Y. 1995. "Photoaging from an Oxidative Point." *Journal of Dermatological Science.* 9:79.

Miyachi, Y., et al. 1988. "The Cumulative Effect of Continual Oxidative Stress to the Skin and Cutaneous Aging." In: *Cutaneous Aging.* A. Kligman and Y. Takase, eds. pp. 435–447, University of Tokyo Press, Tokyo.

Moysan, A., Morquis, I., et al. 1993. "Ultraviolet A-Induced Lipid Peroxidation and Antioxidant Defense Systems in Cultured Human Skin Fibroblasts." *Journal of Investigative Dermatology.* 100:692.

O'Dell, B., et al. 1980. "Diminished Immune Response in Sun-Damaged Skin." *Archives of Dermatology.* 116:559.

Pathak, M. 1987. "Sunscreens and Their Use in the Preventative Treatment of Sunlight-Induced Skin Damage." *Journal of Dermatologic Surgery and Oncology.* 13:739.

Tyrrell, R. 1995. "Ultraviolet Radiation and Free Radical Damage to the Skin." *Biochemical Society Symposia.* 61:47.

Chapter Sixteen: Looking Good Tools II: Diet and Supplements

Black, H., Herd, J., et al. 1994. "Effect of a Low-Fat Diet on the Incidence of Actinic Keratosis." *New England Journal of Medicine.* 330:1272.

Dunn, L., et al. 1997. "Does Estrogen Prevent Skin Aging?" *Archives of Dermatology.* 133:339.

Freyer, M. 1993. "Evidence for the Photoprotective Effects of Vitamin E." *Photochemistry and Photobiology.* 58:304.

Goldfarb, M., Ellis, C., et al. 1990. "Topical Tretinoin: Its Use in Daily Practice to Reverse Photoageing." *British Journal of Dermatology.* 122(suppl. 35):87.

Kligman, A. 1989. "The Treatment of Photoaged Human Skin by Topical Tretinoin." *Drugs.* 38:1.

Matthews-Roth, M., Pathak, M., et al. 1970. "Beta Carotene as a Photoprotective agent in Erythropoietic Protoporphyria." *New England Journal of Medicine.* 282(22):1231.

Matthews-Roth, M., Pathak, M., et al. 1972. "A Clinical Trial of the Effects of Oral Beta Carotene on the Responses of Human Skin to Solar Radiation." *Journal of Investigative Dermatology.* 59(4):349.

Matthews-Roth, M. 1986. "Carotenoids Quench Evolution on Excited Species in Epidermis Exposed to UV-B (290–320 nM) Light." *Photochemistry and Photobiology.* 43:91.

Richard, M., et al. 1993. "Effect of Zinc Supplementation of Resistance of Cultured Human Skin Fibroblasts Towards Oxidant Stress." *Biological Trace Element Research.* 37(2–3):187.

Slaga, T. 1995. "Inhibtion of Skin Tumor Initiation, Promotion, and Progression, by Antioxidants and Related Compounds." *Critical Reviews in Food Science and Nutrition.* 35(1–2):51.

Vahlquist, A., and B. Berne. 1986. "Sunlight, Vitamin A, and the Skin." *Photodermatology.* 3:203.

Index

259

Folate/folic acid, 105-7
Food and Drug Administration (FDA):
  Anafranil, approval of, 204
  food supplements, regulation of, 201
  Halcion, approval of, 205
  L-tryptophan, ban on, 203-4, 205
  melatonin, possible classification as prescription drug, 205
  Prozac, approval of, 204
  regulated industry, relationship with, 201-209
Food supplements, FDA regulation of, 201
Free radicals, 26-27, 88
  cell membrane, damage to, 24-25
  oxygen free radicals. *See* Oxygen free radicals
Free radical theory of aging, 18-20

G
Garlic, benefits of, 173, 205
GH. *See* Growth hormone (GH)
Gingko biloba, 67-70
Glutathione (GSH), 97-99
Glycolic acid. *See* Alpha hydroxy acid
Growth hormone (GH), 137-39
GSH. *See* Glutathione (GSH)
Guided imagery, 189

H
Halcion, FDA approval of, 205
High blood pressure. *See* Hypertension
Holistic medicine, 45, 50-52
Hormone-replacement therapy (HRT), 6, 8, 125, 126-28, 180
  baseline hormone levels, 128
  DHEA. *See* DHEA
  dosage charts. *See* Dosage charts
  estrogen. *See* Estrogen hormone-replacement therapy (EHRT)
  growth hormone, 137-39
  melatonin, 139-44
  testosterone-hormone-replacement therapy. *See* Testosterone-hormone-replacement therapy (THRT)
Hormones, 5, 6
  estrogen, 178-83
  hormone-replacement therapy (HRT). *See* Hormone-replacement therapy (HRT)
  testosterone, 183-86
HRT. *See* Hormone-replacement therapy (HRT)
Hydergine, 63, 71-72
Hypertension:
  physical exercise and, 148

I
Ibuprofen, 114
Immune system, 5, 28-29
  nervous system and, 49
  physical exercise and, 152-53
  stress and, 46, 48, 86
Immune system economics, 86

Iron, 174-75
  Fenton reaction, 174
Iron-deficiency anemia, 174

L
L-deprenyl, 7
Lifespan, 2-3
L-tryptophan, FDA ban on, 203-4, 205
Lucidril. *See* Centrophenoxine (CPH)

M
Massage, 45
Meclofenoxate. *See* Centrophenoxine (CPH)
Meditation, 45, 50, 119-21
  mantra, 121
  resources, 121
  serene mind, 120
Melatonin, 139-44, 201, 202
  FDA's possible classification as prescription drug, 205
  foods high in, 139-44, 143
Memory loss, 64
Mental attitude, 188-89
  "Can't do" attitude, 124
  feeling sexy, 177-78
  feeling young, 177
  guided imagery, 189
  thinking young, 53-54
  visualization, 45, 189-93
Mental exercises, 42, 53, 189-93
Mind exercises. *See* Mental exercises
Motrin, 115
Muscle atrophy, 125

N
Nervous system
  immune system and, 49
  stress and, 47-48
Non-antioxidants:
  antiinflammatories, 114-16
  fatty acids, 109
  folate/folic acid, 105-7
  Omega-3 fatty acids, 109, 111-13
  phosphatidylcholine (PPC), 110-11
  phospholipids, 109
  selenium, 104-5
  zinc, 107-8
Non-sterodial antiinflammatory drugs. *See* Antiinflammatories
Nootropics, 6, 66-67
  acetyl-L-carnitine (ALC), 70-71
  centrophenoxine (CPH), 75-76
  dosage charts, 56-57
  Gingko biloba, 67-70
  Hydergine, 71-72
  naturally occurring, 67
  phosphatidylserine (PPS), 72-73
  Piracetam, 74-75
  synthetic, 73-74
Nuprin, 115

O
Obesity, 159-60
Omega-3 fatty acids, 109, 111-13